DIRT
AND
DISEASE

Polio before FDR

D0069535

Naomi Rogers

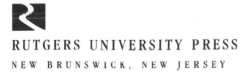

RUTGERS UNIVERSITY PRESS

NEW BRUNSWICK, NEW JERSEY

Library of Congress Cataloging-in-Publication Data

Rogers, Naomi, 1958–
    Dirt and disease : polio before FDR / Naomi Rogers.
      p. cm.—(Health and medicine in American society)
    Includes bibliographical references and index.
    ISBN 0-8135-1785-0 (cloth)—ISBN 0-8135-1786-9 (pbk.)
    1. Poliomyelitis—United States—History. I. Title. II. Series.
    [DNLM: 1. Poliomyelitis—history—United States. WC 555
R728d]
  RA644.P0R64   1990
  614.5′49′0973—dc20
  DNLM/DLC
  for Library of Congress   91-32642
                                               CIP

British Cataloging-in-Publication information available

Dirt and Disease

HEALTH AND MEDICINE
IN AMERICAN SOCIETY
series editors
Judith Walzer Leavitt
Morris Vogel

For my mother, June Factor, my grandmother, Mary Factor, and in memory of my grandfather, Saul Factor

Contents

Acknowledgments   ix

Introduction   1

ONE   Garden of Germs: Polio in the United States,
           1900–1920   9

TWO   This Dread Spectre: Polio and the New Public Health   30

THREE   The Promise of Science: Polio and the Laboratory   72

FOUR   Written in Haste: Polio and the Public   106

FIVE   A Humble and Contrite Frame of Mind: Polio and
           Epidemiology   138

Epilogue   Polio Since FDR   165

Notes   191

Bibliographic Essay   241

Index   249

Acknowledgments

My interest in polio was first stirred by *I Can Jump Puddles* (1955), the autobiography of Alan Marshall, who, as a boy in the Australian bush, had his legs paralyzed by polio in the early 1900s. His unsentimental story of overcoming tremendous obstacles made me think about human resilience and the relations between disease and society. My study dwells more on the social response to polio epidemics than it does on individual experience, but it cannot be understood without acknowledging the strength and determination of the victims of polio and their families.

Researching this work was aided by many archivists and reference librarians. I am grateful to the staffs of the Van Pelt Library of the University of Pennsylvania; the Philadelphia City Archives; the Municipal Archives of New York City; the New York Public Library and its Annex in New York City; the New York Academy of Medicine in New York City; the Rockefeller Archive Center in Tarrytown, New York; the New York State Archives in Albany, New York; the New Jersey State Archives and Library in Trenton, New Jersey; and the libraries of Brown University and the University of Alabama. I am grateful for the special efforts of Beth Carroll-Horrocks of the Manuscripts Room at the American Philosophical Society in Philadelphia; and the staffs at the Reading Room and the Historical Collections at the College of Physicians of Philadelphia, especially Jean Carr and Tom Horrocks.

The structure and approach of this study owes much to my graduate advisor, Charles Rosenberg. He taught me to value the thoughts and experiences of both doctors and patients, and his commitment to scholarship has been an example to me. Michael Katz gave me encouragement throughout my graduate training and helped me remember the broad social and political context of polio in America. Various seminars and academic meetings have sharpened my thoughts on the history of medicine and disease, in particular the Francis C. Wood Institute for the History of Medicine in Philadelphia; the American Association for the History of Medicine annual meetings; the Institute for Health, Health Care Policy, and Aging Research at Rutgers University; the Brown University History seminars; and the Alabama History of Medicine and Science Group.

The generous comments and criticisms of a number of people have helped me rethink this work. I would like to thank especially Hughes Evans, Gina Feldberg, Mary Fissell, Gerald Grob, Alisa Klaus, Harry Marks, Jennifer McClure, Jim Patterson, Joan Richards, Jane Sewell, and Maarten Ultee. Judith Leavitt, Morris Vogel, and Marlie Wasserman, my editors at Rutgers University Press, helped me turn a manuscript into a book, and I am also grateful for the comments of the anonymous reviewer for the Press. Working on this project was made easier and more joyful by the support and encouragement of Rena Bidney, Jo and Danny Burnstein, Mary Murrey, Sue Lederer, Sybil Lipschultz, and especially Lisa Mae Robinson and John Harley Warner who were there when I needed them.

This work bears the imprint of not only my academic training but also my experience as the daughter of an immigrant family. My family in Melbourne provided me with emotional, intellectual, and financial support—the combination that every graduate student and young historian needs. I dedicate this work to my grandmother, Mary Factor, to the memory of my grandfather, Saul Factor, and to my mother, June Factor, my first and most demanding critic, whose love of history, literature, and folklore strengthens my understanding of the past and explains why this work contains poems and stories as well as charts.

Dirt and Disease

Introduction

For most Americans over the age of fifty the word polio has certain consistent images: a smiling freckled girl on crutches on a March of Dimes can; swimming pools closed for the summer; a nurse leaning over a child in an iron lung; rows of children with arms outstretched waiting for their polio vaccine shot; and President Roosevelt seated by a radio microphone, crippled yet strong, America's first handicapped president who refused to allow the press to report his wheelchair, leg braces, or inability to walk.

But before Franklin Roosevelt reached national prominence as either governor of New York or president of the United States, the popular picture of polio was quite different. Polio was associated with the poorest, dirtiest children, not affluent adults in the prime of life, and with immigrants in slums, not Yankees from long-established families. Nor were there iron lungs, or March of Dimes cans, or closed swimming pools. The images we hold are historically specific; they define a particular moment of the disease.

By the late 1920s Roosevelt's paralysis had drawn a wide public awareness of polio. Before this, polio seemed a new and unusual illness. Cases of infantile paralysis, as it was popularly known, were reported occasionally in the nineteenth century; only since the 1890s did epidemics with hundreds and then thousands of victims begin to occur. First reported in isolated towns in Scandinavia in the 1880s and 1890s, polio epidemics had by 1920 troubled not only Sweden, Norway, and the United States but also France, England, Germany, and Australia, and they were increasingly an urban as well as a rural health problem. From the outset, the disease did not appear to be restricted to children from a single group: it attacked children of all classes, from both slums and suburbs. As well, its spread seemed random; often only one member of a family or a street block was paralyzed while siblings and neighboring children were left untouched.

Polio was not a new disease, but its appearance in epidemic form was new. Before the 1890s nonparalytic polio was endemic and rarely recognized or recorded. Most children were infected by the polio virus through maternal antibodies or as infants. This early infection usually produces only a mild fever and then lifelong immunity. But, like measles, polio infection is most dangerous when it occurs among those who have developed no immunity in infancy. If children, protected from the virus, are infected at a later age, they are more likely to develop the paralytic symptoms we call "polio," as the virus spreads from the intestines to the nervous system. In the twentieth century, as more children in industrialized Western countries were protected from disease through improved sanitation and childcare, diseases such as cholera and typhoid began to decline, but polio cases grew. Thus, by 1900, while most poor immigrant children had become infected and immune at an early age, children from clean, middle-class homes were at greater risk of the paralytic form of the disease. The danger of epidemic polio did not diminish until the development of effective polio vaccines in the 1950s. Since the widespread use of vaccines over the past three decades, polio has rarely appeared in epidemic form in developed countries, although it remains both endemic and epidemic in countries with inadequate sanitation, nutrition, and medical resources.

Until the 1930s and 1940s little of this was known. Nonetheless scientists continued to study polio's pathology, physicians debated possible therapies and causes, and the public faced potential epidemics with fear and dread. This study examines the early years of epidemic polio in the United States from 1900 to 1920. By examining how one disease was defined I explore the ways scientific medicine shaped and was shaped by American society and culture. Polio epidemics highlighted tensions between old and new medical theories and practices, as physicians, scientists, and the lay public debated the increasing authority of scientific medicine. After 1921 the meaning and significance of polio shifted, as the disease began to take on its new image as "Roosevelt's disease."

Recent experience with AIDS has heightened our awareness of the significance of the social meanings of an epidemic, the powerful metaphoric link between dirt and disease, and the sanctions imposed on those groups believed to be spreading infection. Defining and assigning responsibility is an essential element in making sense of an epidemic. The case of polio is distinctive and its early history in the United States ironic, for, although we now link the disease with cleanliness, cases among middle-class native-born families were then interpreted as anomalous. And efforts to prevent the spread of the disease centered on instructing families in proper hygiene and childcare.

The years that polio epidemics first appeared in the United States were also the high point of the new scientific medicine and the germ theory. Physicians and the lay public hoped that new techniques drawn from the work of European scientists Louis Pasteur and Robert Koch would transform the social landscape and conquer diseases that regularly plagued many communities. The most potent symbol of scientific medicine was the laboratory whose products offered physicians new ways to diagnose, treat, and prevent disease. But, in this period, the problem of polio was not resolved by placing the laboratory at the center of medical and public health practice.

In their frustrating inability to explain or control epidemic polio, scientists, physicians, and the public looked for groups to blame. Health officials, focusing their work on immigrant families who had recently arrived from Southern and Eastern Europe, claimed that the unsanitary habits of these families had spread the disease from tenement slums to the homes of more careful middle-class citizens. Using the ideology of scientific medicine, proponents of a new movement in public health admitted that, in theory, germs could randomly spread disease across ethnic, class, and racial lines and that moral behavior, other than in strict sanitary ways, would not protect an individual from infection. Assumptions that poor immigrants through carelessness and ignorance were spreading polio, however, were strong enough to overcome the gradual intellectual changes that public health theory and practice had undergone since the 1890s. Furthermore, health officials' concern with the physical environment in their efforts to guard health reflected the continuing nineteenth-century beliefs that linked moral to physical health and cleanliness to social order.

In the Progressive era, the period from 1890 to 1920, American physicians and scientists struggled to become the accepted experts in guiding health care and health policy. Science, they argued, would bring objectivity as well as efficiency to public health work. The solutions proposed by the new experts were largely oriented around changing the behavior of individuals. As health officials guarded the community's health by keeping food, water, and streets clean, disease became a sign of individual irresponsibility, a failure to carry out the well understood rules of modern hygiene. Reformers assumed that even the immigrant poor were able to control their sanitary conditions and domestic health. The irony of the polio story is that health experts targeted just those homes in which children were likely to be already immune.

Yet the introduction and gradual popularization of the germ theory of disease in the 1880s and 1890s and the spectacular successes of bacteriology had clouded the issue of responsibility for illness. Germs appeared sometimes in filth but sometimes insidiously in those who seemed clean and healthy. Medical professionals and the lay public nonetheless hoped that careful bacteriological investigation could answer troublesome questions about the spread of epidemic disease. To explain polio they also turned to the new science of medical entomology. Polio cases that appeared in the suburbs, among families of wealth and substance, could have suggested a link between the disease and cleanliness, but officials sought other explanations. An anti-fly campaign that portrayed flies as carrying the disease from working-class to middle-class homes was especially powerful and successful.

This study explores the American experience of epidemic polio from a number of perspectives. My focus is specifically on the epidemic of 1916, the most serious polio epidemic the United States had ever experienced. During its brief five-month appearance the epidemic starkly illuminated urban life. Governors and mayors exhorted health officials and medical experts to police polio victims and possible carriers and (reminiscent of earlier times) granted local health boards extraordinary quarantine powers. Hotelkeepers in resort towns, managers of movie theaters, directors of railroad companies, and customers in department stores all called for a way to identify people and objects that might spread the disease.

Polio research was conducted in laboratories run by state and municipal health authorities and the private Rockefeller Institute for Medical Research in New York City. Polio investigators had to be familiar with a complex and contradictory literature, and their use of monkeys as laboratory animals made research more expensive and difficult. Private physicians and members of the public saw these scientists as authoritative experts, although their efforts to develop methods to diagnose and treat polio were disappointingly inadequate. The most promising work on polio that combined field and laboratory studies was based on the methods of epidemiology, still a fledging discipline professionally and intellectually. But this integration proved as difficult as controlling the disease. Epidemiological studies of polio, largely shaped by nineteenth-century models of health reform, remained focused on the conditions of working-class and immigrant homes. Filth, poverty, and overcrowding had successfully predicted other infectious infant diseases, but they did not explain the distribution of polio cases. Indeed, suburban and rural areas often had a higher proportion of polio cases than crowded slums; this suggested that cleanliness might facilitate the spread of the disease. But American epidemiologists, despite the evidence of their fieldwork, refused to take this intellectual leap of faith.

In this study I particularly stress the social history of polio. Public health efforts to explain and control polio grew out of the differing experiences and expectations of those who encountered the disease. Anti-polio campaigns were negotiated between health officials and the lay public. Health officials tried to use modern methods of science to calm the public and halt the spread of the disease, but they returned to the familiar public health litany of quarantine and sanitation. Some families resisted official efforts to blame them; others responded by locking their children indoors, even in the summer heat, to protect them from other possibly infected children and from breathing infected air. During the 1916 epidemic letters written to medical experts by members of the public suggest that the new sciences were considered a public resource, in vocabulary and metaphor, as well as an object of criticism. Scientific medicine was becoming a familiar, yet not the only, way to explain sickness, nor had it fully replaced traditional explanations of the cause of disease and the workings of the body.

American popular and professional responses to epidemic polio in the 1900s and 1910s illustrate the continuing power of belief about the relations between dirt, disease, and disorder. The germ theory and the new scientific medicine did not magically dissipate the influence of cultural prejudice in defining the relationship among disease, environment, and individual behavior. Indeed, in this era, polio epidemics highlighted the limitations of scientific solutions to social and political problems.

Since this period, the public has demonstrated a growing faith in scientific authority. Yet the tensions between scientific reductionism and civic responsibility have been raised with special urgency in recent years. In the mid-1980s many American gay rights advocates, pinning their hopes on the development of a vaccine, rejected broad explanations of the role of moral and sexual behavior in defining AIDS. Yet gay activists have in the past sought to engage with community mores; in the 1970s sexual freedom had become a hallmark of gay identity. Conservative critics, by contrast, have argued that the AIDS epidemic is the emergence, in a concrete and deadly form, of the social and cultural decay of our modern society. For them, harsh environmental measures—such as testing and labeling high-risk groups, instituting quarantine measures, and denying employment—are appropriate ways to assuage public fear and hysteria and punish the victims assumed guilty. The hopes of both sides reflect the established authority of the laboratory as a means for preventing disease, curing the sick, and identifying carriers. Faith in laboratory research reinforces a belief in the transforming power of scientific understanding. Controversy over whether and how to instruct the public about safe sex also reflects the long-standing belief by many health experts that altering an individual's personal behavior can protect the community's health.

The fear of dirt and its association with disease persists into our own world. This study suggests that explanations of the workings of disease have underlying social and political ideologies, sometimes only made explicit in times of urgency, such as an epidemic. The long-held connection between dirt and disease did not just disappear with widespread knowledge of the germ theory. It continues to hold a powerful intellectual and practical appeal: it combines morality and science; it helps to distinguish rich from poor, native-born from immigrant, the ignorant and careless from the informed and responsible. Perhaps with a disease as challenging to traditional epidemiological patterns as epidemic polio these connections became an even stronger part of public health rhetoric.

The paradox of epidemic polio was not resolved in the early twentieth century. Clearly it involved the whole community, yet particular groups were singled out for special attention and attack. The new sciences provided standards and vocabulary to aid these efforts, but their experts could neither offer objective, effective means to control nor explain the spread of the disease. This study, then, stands in contrast to any notion that science and its voice alone can solve our social problems. In fact, there is not one voice of science but many. To explain polio, laboratory workers, physicians, officials, and the public debated and interpreted the methods and concepts of science. A fear of dirt and immigrants played an important part in helping them identify the guilty and the innocent. Integrating the germ theory did not solve the problem of determining responsibility for disease. Some groups were still believed more culpable than others.

CHAPTER ONE

Garden of Germs: Polio in the United States, 1900–1920

In 1917 Manton M. Carrick, a reform-minded Texas physician, came to New York City and paid a visit to the American Museum of Natural History. Writing later in a women's magazine, Carrick remarked on a new addition to the museum's famed "Garden of Germs." A new germ had just been added to the seven hundred already displayed in a glass case: the polio germ.

Polio, Carrick noted, was not a new disease, for it had appeared sporadically since the early 1800s, but recently it had become a serious menace. After members of his community in Texas had read about New York City's struggles against polio a year earlier, they had conducted a "preparedness" campaign. "Inasmuch as we brush against people of all classes continually in trolleys, elevators and shops it seems rather dangerous for us to neglect the localities in which they live," Carrick reflected, for "disease is not always a respecter of persons, as Poliomyelitis and other epidemics have proven to us." The best weapon to use against polio, he argued, was cleanliness, "a thoroughgoing campaign against dirt in every nook and corner." He and his fellow reformers had sought to "awaken civic pride and to educate people as to their rights." They proceeded, therefore, to clean parks, streets and alleys, insane asylums, jails, orphanages, and slums. The campaign against polio included fly-swatting contests for children, boycotts by housewives of grocers, butchers, and bakers who had not properly cleaned their stores, and other methods of popular education. Carrick also strongly recommended *Fighting Infantile Paralysis,* a motion picture that had been produced with the assistance of the Rockefeller Institute for Medical Research. This film he wrote,

> not only depicts the horror of the disease, but is constructively educational. The scenes show narrow streets lined with dirty and unsanitary pushcarts, the latter filled with fly-specked cakes and candy and decaying fruit, all are touched by many hands before they are finally eaten; there are uncovered garbage cans near which cats and children play and squabble over crusts of bread and other tid-bits; the Street Department taking care of its garbage and flushing its streets; the course taken by infantile paralysis from the moment the germ invades the spinal cord and brain via the blood, to the last stage when the disabled patient is compelled to take after-treatment.[1]

This description neatly captures many issues raised by epidemic polio in early twentieth-century urban America: disease was linked to both dirt and immigrants who came into contact with native-born middle-class Americans; municipal health officers worked as both sanitary regulators and popular educators; scientists searched for the polio germ in the laboratory; and physicians tried to heal the sick and disabled.

Americans in the early 1900s saw the sudden appearance of what seemed to be a new epidemic disease. Poliomyelitis paralyzed infants and children. Their economic or sanitary conditions seemed to make little difference; rich or poor, clean or dirty, no child seemed immune. Polio epidemics appeared in most Western nations, but the disease was a peculiarly American problem. Between 1905 and 1909, according to one report, of eight thousand polio cases reported worldwide, almost two-thirds had appeared in the United States.[2]

This study is based primarily around the American response to the 1916 epidemic. In 1916 the United States witnessed the world's then largest polio epidemic: 27,000 cases and 6,000 deaths in twenty-six states. Between June and December in New

York City alone there were 8,900 cases and 2,400 deaths, a mortality rate of around one child in four.

Early in the summer of 1916 mothers began coming to infant health stations in Brooklyn, carrying paralyzed children in their arms. Nurses at the stations were at a loss: What could they do? The children had routine clinical histories: they had developed stomach trouble or diarrhea, become feverish, restless, or irritable, and then awakened the next morning unable to move an arm or leg.[3]

Soon these children were of more than local interest; their symptoms were identified as "infantile paralysis," the popular term for polio. By mid-June these New York cases had turned into an epidemic, and in early July the city's mayor expanded the emergency powers of the public health department by declaring New York formally in a "state of peril."[4] The epidemic appeared to have originated in Brooklyn, before spreading to other New York City boroughs, then the neighboring states of New Jersey, Pennsylvania, and Connecticut, and along the eastern seaboard generally. In July more than seven hundred cases and one hundred deaths were reported in New York City; this equaled the total number for the entire last major northeastern epidemic of 1907. Although there were some cases reported in Ohio, Rhode Island, Kansas, Wisconsin, and Illinois, the epidemic became clearly a problem for the mid-Atlantic states. The U.S. Public Health Service sent epidemiologists and bacteriologists to investigate the epidemic, and by mid-August federal health officers reported that New York State had 6,653 cases, New Jersey 1,740, and Pennsylvania and Connecticut more than 300.[5] Health officials responded by establishing state quarantines and trying to identify and isolate cases. Physicians and scientists met regularly in a series of conferences to discuss methods of prevention, treatment, and control—but to little avail. The epidemic peaked in August, and with the cooler fall weather cases gradually declined.[6] In early September health officials lifted their restrictions on public gatherings, and schools opened only a few weeks later than usual; by October most quarantine placards had been taken down, and the U.S. Public Health Service officials had returned to Washington.[7]

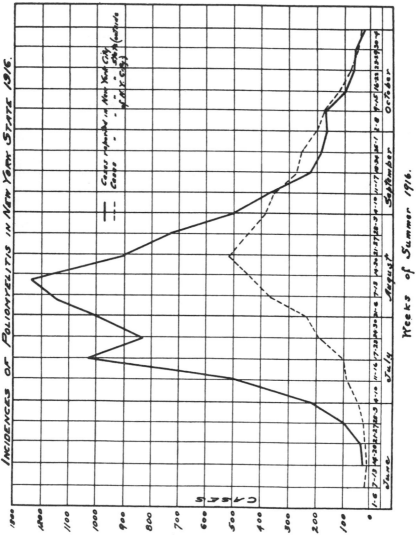

Fig. 1 The rise and fall of the 1916 epidemic in New York City and State

The shape of the 1916 epidemic can only be partly uncovered, for historians have been left with evidence limited by the categories and assumptions of contemporary investigators. The researchers who studied the epidemic judged certain factors relevant and left out others. Early in the epidemic they expected to find that race and ethnicity would play an important role in explaining polio's spread, reflected by the design of cards for special investigations. But when they found cases among both immigrant and native-born middle-class children they decided that ethnicity was a largely irrelevant epidemiological variable. Similarly, because so few black children were reported, some researchers began to debate the idea of a racial immunity to polio; race thus became invisible in most later studies.[8] Cases and deaths were higher among males than females, a difference also unexplained but not unusual for other diseases.[9] The factor of age was considered important. Epidemic polio was clearly a children's disease; in New York City and Newark around 80 percent of cases were under five years old. The most critical distinguishing factor was the differences noted between rural and urban areas. Polio victims in rural counties in New York State were older than urban children and more likely to die. New York City officials also found a higher proportion of cases in Queens and Staten Island than in densely populated Manhattan.[10] These figures reflect not only the widespread immunity among adults in urban and congested areas but also the endemic mild cases of polio missed by most physicians; these ideas were debated at the time but not integrated into most analyses of the epidemic. The notion that dirt could protect a child from disease was thoroughly alien to all conventional etiological explanations of the workings of disease, and contemporary researchers did not consider that possibility. In any case, they sought more immediate practical ways to explain and control the epidemic.

For a brief time, polio became part of America's national culture. Cartoonists used the disease to symbolize politics, baseball, and war. The metaphor of invasion had immediate resonance in 1916, for the European war had taken over the front pages of most major newspapers, and the Democratic and Republican party conventions were relegated to inner pages.[11] Fighting infection, wrote one New York physician, depended on the "virulence of the aggressor." "Here," he continued, "there is no place for pacifists, piece [sic]-at-any-price plans or unpreparedness." Another doctor urged health officials to put up banners like those at recent preparedness parades across streets in "the thickly populated districts where the disease is prevalent" to warn of the dangers of recklessness in breaking simple hygienic rules.[12] Local measures against polio were on occasion described in these terms. New York summer travelers complained that in some New Jersey communities they were treated "like European refugees fleeing before drives and counter-drives of the contending armies."[13]

Polio appeared particularly strange and frightening because of physicians' and the public's high expectations of science and scientists. By 1909 the etiological agent of polio had been established as a virus, but bacteria and viruses were only vaguely differentiated. For decades polio remained only partially understood and difficult to treat, prevent, or even diagnose.

The confusion surrounding polio struck a jarring note in this time of scientific optimism. The period from 1890 to 1920 has been termed "the age of scientific medicine," the beginning of a new era in medical practice and research. New techniques of bacteriology and pathology developed in the 1870s and 1880s by European scientists Louis Pasteur and Robert Koch were integrated into medical practice and popularized in the lay community through displays such as the Museum of Natural History's Garden of Germs.

The appeal to scientific expertise and faith in transforming individual behavior were touchstones for reformers during this Progressive era. As they attacked corrupt urban machines, inequitable corporate business practices, and the working conditions of the urban poor, Progressive reformers increasingly relied on professional, university-trained experts whose work would, they believed, transform the city into a clean, pleasant, and efficient place. The groups believed most important to educate in the values of expertise and efficiency were immigrants from Southern and Eastern Europe who were flooding American cities.

This reform work, which included establishing model kitchens, settlement houses, and baby welfare stations, was based on a faith in popular education. It targeted women in particular, for, as housekeepers and homemakers, they were the guardians of the family's spiritual and physical health. Reformers hoped that, by teaching the public the lessons of science, they would inspire families to change their habits of hygiene and nutrition and so protect themselves, their homes, and their communities.[14] Carrick's "preparedness" campaign reflected both reformers' assumptions about the link between cleanliness and social order and the need for civic-minded experts to regulate public and private space.

The appearance of a frightening new disease just as scientists were conquering the old seemed strange and inappropriate. Polio epidemics also contradicted traditional models of disease transmission: polio cases appeared in both overcrowded slums and sparsely populated suburbs; they attacked not only Italian and Russian families but also assimilated Germans, Irish, and the native-born. Its victims were often children who were previously healthy, well nourished, and protected. Campaigns against the uneducated and the careless did not make sense if the dirty were not the guilty victims and carriers of disease.

POLIO AND PUBLIC HEALTH

In 1920 the germ theory was only about a generation old. Most American physicians had been trained at medical schools that espoused the filth theory of disease and taught students through didactic lectures rather than the clinical and laboratory experience advocated by Paris clinicians and German researchers. During their working lives, however, American practitioners had witnessed the identification of specific causative agents of diseases, including diphtheria, tuberculosis, cholera, typhoid, and syphilis. Increasingly, physicians had come to see disease as a specific, distinct process rather than a shifting protean condition whose development and treatment depended on the patient's individual characteristics.

In the decades after the Civil War, health departments that had been established to deal with epidemic emergencies assumed sanitary responsibilities such as garbage disposal, street cleaning, and food regulation.[15] The filth theory of disease provided the intellectual basis for this public health work.[16] The filth theory and its public health practice, sanitary science, were, however, gradually undermined by the successes of bacteriologic research in the 1880s and 1890s and the development of specific, laboratory-based techniques for identifying and combating disease agents. The promoters of this New Public Health expected that professionally trained health experts would identify germs, develop sera and vaccines, and instruct individuals in the values of scientific medicine and their responsibility for the prevention of disease. These new attitudes shifted public health work from an environmentally grounded view of health and sickness to a behavioral one in which the habits of individuals became a major focus of health policy.[17]

One singular champion of this new approach was Charles V. Chapin, health officer of Providence, Rhode Island. Chapin, fervently rejecting sanitary science, believed that the germ theory and the discoveries of bacteriologists should be integrated into public health work. He discouraged the use of older public health measures like disinfection, fumigation, and public sanitation; a dirty city, he argued, could be a healthy city. Officials should instead begin identifying and treating human carriers, using the laboratory rather than the broom or water filter as a public health instrument.[18] By the 1890s Chapin had transformed the Providence health department into a model of his ideas. Health professionals from all over North America came to view the department's laboratory, its increasing use of medically trained personnel, and its extensive regulatory and educational programs. In New York and other states health officials began to adopt Chapin's approach.[19]

Chapin's arguments spurred the changes public health departments were already experiencing during the Progressive era. By the 1910s most American health officials worked in a new intellectual and institutional context. Nineteenth-century officials had usually been part-time reformers with a concern for their community's environment, and most major urban health boards were run by a collection of public-spirited elite citizens interested in sanitation and reform. By 1916 most urban officials worked in newly professionalized, municipally funded health departments staffed by medically trained experts.[20]

The transformation of public health departments was reinforced by Progressive reformers. During previous generations urban public health departments had wielded only limited and temporary power; they were now established permanently with expansive regulatory powers. Progressive reformers, trying to remake the character of city departments as well as their powers, sought to change them from their position as graft-ridden cogs of urban political machines to efficient and fair organizations run by university trained experts. Although in some parts of city hall the impact of these efforts was difficult for contemporaries to assess, health officials found that applying the methods of science could dramatically improve the public's health. Bacteriology had proven especially rewarding; it made visible specific agents of disease in water, food, and blood and provided physicians with precise tests to identify the microorganisms of various diseases, including the Widal test for typhoid, the Schick for diphtheria, and the Wassermann for syphilis. Physicians and health officials grew increasingly confident that epidemics would be conquered with the knowledge of the mechanism of disease transmission, the laboratory diagnosis of germs, and the use of sera and vaccines. "The bacteriologist," wrote a contemporary, "bending over the microscope and culture tube in the quiet laboratory, stands between death and the children."[21]

The introduction of bacteriological methods into public health work provided officials with new weapons for dealing with disease. By 1920 many health departments had in their arsenals a number of diagnostic and therapeutic tools based on the germ theory. New York State's public health laboratories produced vaccines against smallpox, rabies, whooping cough, and typhoid, sera for dysentery, meningitis, and pneumonia, and antitoxins for diphtheria and tetanus. New York City physicians could draw on the city's public health laboratory for diagnostic tests for tuberculosis, gonorrhea, malaria, typhoid, diphtheria, syphilis,

and rabies.[22] Many doctors hoped that the application of laboratory techniques to health problems would help direct methods of
disease control, therapy, and diagnosis and ultimately provide
the knowledge and tools to conquer sickness and transform the
social landscape. Yet the contemporary experience of syphilis—a
disease with both a diagnostic test and effective therapy—had
shown that such solutions were not so straightforward. Cases of
venereal disease continued to increase, and efforts at popular
education about the disease were entangled with social mores of
sexuality and morality.[23]

Although these laboratory products were potent symbols of
the promise of laboratory science, polio epidemics appeared
during an era of transition in the American public health movement. Promoters of the New Public Health urged the public to
accept the germ theory, but the popular and professional association between dirt and disease lingered. Officials sought to
make germs as fearful as filth, but, unlike garbage and overflow-
ing sewers, germs were not readily visible. Sanitary science had
offered pragmatic ways for officials to show communities that
their health was being protected; the germ theory promoted by
the New Public Health seemed less intuitively compelling.[24]
Flushing streets and disinfecting buildings were dramatic methods of guarding a community's health, but killing germs did not
provide such dramatic opportunities.

Officials who sought to integrate these conflicting conceptions
of public health theory and practice found that one resolution to
the contradictions involved promoting the idea that insects
spread disease. Work by Ronald Ross in malaria and Walter Reed
in yellow fever had demonstrated that germs could be spread by
insects; the campaigns against both the yellow fever mosquito
while building the Panama Canal and the hookworm in the
American South and Latin America were impressive signs of
efforts to control disease by eliminating insects.[25] Physicians and
health officials could now offer the public practical ways to attack
filth and at the same time focus on specific etiological agents of
disease. The insect theory explained not only the etiology of a
disease but also the specific mechanism of its transmission. The
familiar insects could be caught and killed by both officials and

housekeepers. Furthermore, most household insects were associated with dirt, overcrowding, and poverty,—these environmental factors continued the link between public health work, urban
reform, and the filth theory of disease.

During the first two decades of this century the housefly was a
favorite target for health officials. Anti-fly crusades exemplified
health reformers' faith in popular education as an important tool
of the New Public Health movement and enabled officials to
demonstrate the implications of bacteriology and entomology
for everyday life. Thus, a careful housekeeper could ensure her
family's health by guarding her home from the housefly. Like
Carrick's description of the 1916 polio film, officials linked sanitary health work with education campaigns that warned of the
dangers (both visible and invisible) of food, filth, and flies as well
as germs.

In their anti-polio campaigns American health officials and
private physicians turned to the laboratory for therapeutic and
diagnostic help. But at the peak of public hysteria they also
relied on tried and true methods of disinfection and fumigation. Despite the measures' contradictions to tenets of the New
Public Health, relying on sanitary regulation was partly the result of the laboratory's impotence in dealing with and explaining polio. Health officials acknowledged that their efforts
against polio were general rather than specific. New York City
Health Commissioner Haven Emerson explained that his department did not enforce sanitary regulations during the 1916
epidemic "with the idea that it would have anything to do with
stopping the spread of the epidemic. We did it with the idea of
taking advantage at this time of public susceptibility and we
considered that the time was favorable to hit hard and try to get
people to obey the law."[26]

Polio proved confusing and intractable to bacteriological, epidemiological, and therapeutic measures of the day. Unable to
offer much effective treatment or preventives to frightened
parents or crippled children, public health officials fell back on
scapegoating immigrant families such as Brooklyn Italians and
Lower East Side Jews. Although anti-fly campaigns could have
targeted the entire community, officials largely blamed the

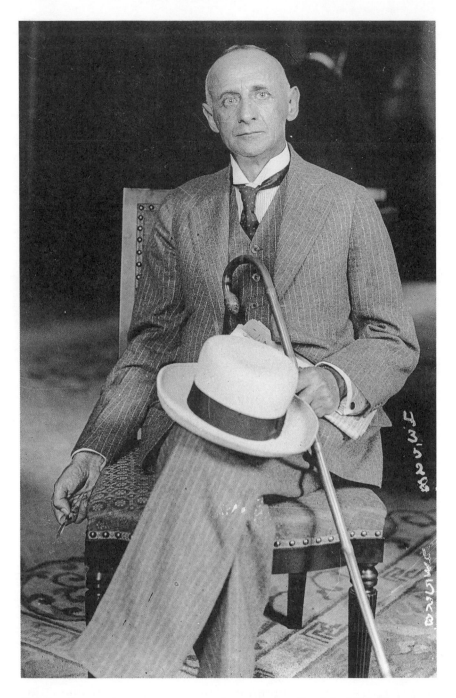

Fig. 2 Simon Flexner at press conference on polio, July 1916 (Bettmann Archives)

spread of polio on immigrants who through ignorance and carelessness carried dangerous germs and flies to the middle-class home.[27] That polio was spread by flies seemed only to justify a belief in the dire results of sanitary irresponsibility and ignorance. Health officials ordered nightly street cleaning in immigrant neighborhoods; and small town communities ordered the "clean-up" of slum districts. The 1916 anti-polio campaign had clear ethnic and class dimensions; officials tried to keep the disease from every door, but when confronted with their own inadequacies, they defined middle- and upper-class families as innocent victims, and poor immigrant families as guilty carriers. Ironically, while the latter lived in unsanitary conditions and certainly faced many contagious diseases, polio was to become an increasing problem for the clean, protected children of the suburbs rather than the slums.

THE STATE OF POLIO SCIENCE

During the height of the 1916 polio epidemic the *New York Times* profiled scientist Simon Flexner. Flexner was already established as a prominent scientific figure in the popular and professional press. Trained at Johns Hopkins Medical School among the nation's outstanding medical researchers, Flexner was a fervent proponent and spokesman of the new scientific medicine.[28] In 1903 he had been appointed the first laboratory director of the Rockefeller Institute for Medical Research, a private research institute established by John D. Rockefeller.[29] Asked about his laboratory studies on polio in 1916, Flexner told reporters confidently that he and his colleague Hideyo Noguchi had managed to see the germ of polio itself, which appeared in the dark microscope as "innumerable bright dancing points, devoid of definite size and form."[30] Perhaps Flexner and Noguchi's "dancing points" were the model for the germ that the Museum of Natural History added to its Garden of Germs.

Private physicians and the public had come to expect this kind of announcement from bacteriologists, particularly Rockefeller scientists. The founding of research institutes in New

York City, Chicago, Philadelphia, and San Francisco reflected a growing interest in scientific research. These institutes, modeled on the Koch Institute in Berlin and the Pasteur Institute in Paris, for the first time offered researchers in the United States the opportunity to work without the added responsibilities of private practice or academic teaching.[31]

From its inception the Rockefeller Institute concentrated on pure scientific research; it was, according to the *New York Times*, full of "scientific men, working in the scientific spirit, and that spirit is not concerned with impressing the multitude."[32] But its directors found that they faced a somewhat suspicious public. In an era when the name Rockefeller was associated with labor disputes and secret trusts, the Institute's quest for public support led its members to engage in a number of local health issues, including the disease-ridden New York milk supply and local epidemics of meningitis and poliomyelitis.[33] Flexner also conducted well-publicized campaigns against the antivivisectionist movement's attempt to restrict the use of animals for experimental research. At times, this led him to exaggerate the promise of science. In 1911, in the heart of a battle against antivivisectionists who were pressuring the New York State legislature, Flexner told the *New York Times* that the cure for polio was not far distant.[34] The Institute, moreover, helped produce the 1916 film *Fighting Infantile Paralysis*, in which scientists and health officials work together to fight the ravages of the disease, with the informed cooperation of the public.

The state of polio research did not inspire much public confidence, largely because scientists were unable to agree on the cause of the disease; nor was the debate about the agent of polio resolved by Flexner's 1916 announcement. In 1908 and 1909 researchers in Vienna and Paris established that polio was caused by an infectious organism that could be cultured in animals. Following Robert Koch's rules of bacteriological proof, Flexner amplified this work, showing that the polio microorganism could be transmitted from experimental monkey to monkey and that the microbe was a special kind: a filterable virus smaller than all known bacteria. Viral agents had already been established for yellow fever, smallpox, and rabies.[35] Today, scientists believe that viruses are not simply small bacteria, but distinct agents that grow and multiply only on living material. In the early twentieth century, however, many investigators agreed with Noguchi that with the proper mixture and technique it was possible to grow any germ.[36] Cultivating the polio virus proved difficult, but in 1913 Flexner and Noguchi, noting a "globoid" shape and other distinctive characteristics, discovered what they believed to be the virus itself.[37] But their cultivation techniques were extremely delicate. Not only did few other researchers manage to obtain similar results, but many were also swayed by competing theories of other polio agents, including a diplococcus and a streptococcus.[38]

The way the virus entered and spread through the body was also unresolved. *Fighting Infantile Paralysis* portrayed a polio microorganism that invaded the brain and spinal cord via the blood, but, even within the Rockefeller Institute, this was not a widely accepted notion of the way the polio virus traveled through the body. Flexner, whose work became virological orthodoxy for the next few decades, argued that the virus traveled through the nerves directly after entering the body; thus, polio was primarily a nerve disease.[39]

Flexner's notion of polio stemmed largely from his laboratory procedures. Because the polio virus was difficult to see, the ability to produce symptoms of paralysis in animals remained one of the most significant ways laboratory workers had to establish the existence and virulence of the virus. Like European researchers Karl Landsteiner and Constanin Levaditi, Flexner chose Rhesus monkeys as his experimental animal. He found that the most effective way to give this species polio was to inject infected material directly into the spine or brain. At autopsy Flexner found significant lesions in the brain and spinal cord; this reinforced the idea that polio was a disease that primarily attacked the nerves. Historian Saul Benison has characterized this early polio research as based on a "pathology of symptoms."[40] The expense and difficulty of keeping and handling monkeys further restricted the institutions able to pursue polio research.

Drawing analogies between a disease in humans and symptoms

in animals is often risky. Flexner's choice of Rhesus monkeys led him to argue that polio was primarily a neurological disease. But Rhesus monkeys, unlike other primate species, can be infected only through injecting the virus into the brain; other species can develop the disease after being fed the virus by mouth, the way most humans are infected.[41] Furthermore, as Flexner passed viral material from monkey to monkey over a series of years, his strain (later known as MV or mixed virus) became neurotropic. That is, unlike most polio viruses in animals and humans, this virus affected only the central nervous system and would not replicate in the intestines, which the infection does naturally; it became a neural-adapted virus.[42] In this sense, Flexner and his colleagues created a virus in the laboratory and then erroneously began to relate its properties to the clinical experience of the disease.

In the pre-antibiotic era it was difficult to ensure sterile laboratory cultures. Scientists today are not surprised that researchers before the 1940s found numerous multishaped forms in test tubes and dishes. It is unclear what these were; one historian has generously suggested that Flexner and Noguchi may have in fact seen faint evidence of polio antibodies.[43] Not until the late 1920s did younger virologists, including Rockefeller scientist Thomas Rivers, begin to publish work that contradicted Flexner's model of polio. By this time Flexner had retired from active research, and Noguchi was dead.[44] Rivers and other young researchers, attacking the idea that Flexner and Noguchi had cultivated polio "globoid bodies," argued that viruses cannot grow in nonliving material. In 1948 Boston virologist John Enders, in work that won him and his research team a Nobel Prize, developed a technique to grow a strain of the polio virus in nonneurological tissue. Significantly he did not use Flexner's standard MV strain.[45] By the 1950s there was a new model of polio as a disease that entered the body through the mouth, traveled to the intestines via the blood, and only on occasion affected the nervous system.

Flexner's polio work shaped the direction of American virology for the rest of the twentieth century. It structured not only subsequent polio research and clinical trials but also other viral research. The polio virus became the virus on which most young American virologists from the 1910s to the 1950s cut their experimental teeth. Moreover, Flexner's conception of laboratory research reinforced the idea that a scientist need not integrate clinical studies; later polio researchers regretted this laboratory-based research agenda.[46]

In the United States most laboratory research on polio during this era was conducted in private institutes or elite universities. Although some health departments pursued original laboratory research, few scientists were employed full-time by health departments other than the U.S. Public Health Service. A survey of forty-seven state boards of health in 1914 found that most used their laboratories to examine water and milk, and only twenty conducted original research. State-funded research tended to be aimed at immediate health problems such as infected food or outbreaks of disease. During 1914, for example, the state board of health of Florida conducted research on the bacterial flora of soda fountain glasses; its counterpart in Kansas studied the problem of spoiled canned food.[47]

By 1916 scientists had developed two bacteriological techniques to try to solve the problems of diagnosing and treating polio. They expanded the use of the spinal tap in order to analyze a polio patient's spinal fluid and developed and tested a polio serum using the blood of recovered polio victims. But despite these tools, the promise of the laboratory remained unfulfilled, and epidemics were frightening and unpredictable. Years after scientists identified the polio virus, newspapers continued to report that the "germ" of polio had not been discovered.[48] While physicians and members of the public increasingly accepted the application of laboratory methods to investigate the workings of disease, they remained uneasy when these methods did not provide clear conclusions. Not surprisingly, the public expressed dissatisfaction with science and scientists during polio epidemics. In 1916 one Philadelphian reflected in a letter to a local newspaper that "the ignorance of the medical profession in this instance is appalling, and is quite sufficient to cause lack of confidence and distrust toward the whole profession."[49]

Elite scientific experts were not the only group concerned

about polio. Local doctors, sanitarians, and health officials, and of course the public, also contributed to the debate. Physicians who wrote to local medical journals offered their experience of one or two cases. Municipal, state, and federal health officials published studies of epidemics.[50] Some polio fighters were career sanitarians and public health workers rather than scientists or private practitioners. Prominent among these was Haven Emerson, a representative of a brief reformist era in city politics, who headed the New York City's Department of Health during the 1916 epidemic. The son of a physician and sanitarian, Emerson combined public health work with temperance reform; he later became professor of preventive medicine at Columbia University.[51] His work reflected a new emphasis on applying the findings of science to society. Interest in preventive medicine during the first two decades of this century had grown as members of the medical profession began to take a forceful role in shaping society's health policies, whether through government or private agencies.[52] This move toward what was later termed social medicine did not always fit neatly with the growing reliance on the laboratory as the first and last medical resort. Among elite scientists, the practical concerns of most general practitioners and social reformers trailed behind more abstract research.[53]

The opening of the Johns Hopkins School of Public Health and Hygiene in 1919 signaled the growing professionalization of American public health. One early public health professional who popularized the idea that flies spread polio was Milton J. Rosenau, author of a major public health textbook, *Preventive Medicine and Hygiene* (1913). In 1909 he left the U.S. Public Health Service to become professor of preventive medicine and hygiene at the Harvard Medical School. He also headed the short-lived joint Harvard-MIT School for Health Officers, which lasted from 1913 until 1922.[54] Other officials who shaped polio health policy were Hermann M. Biggs, commissioner of health for New York State, and Samuel G. Dixon who held a similar position in Pennsylvania. Both were prominent public figures with a broad interest in disease prevention. Bigg's death

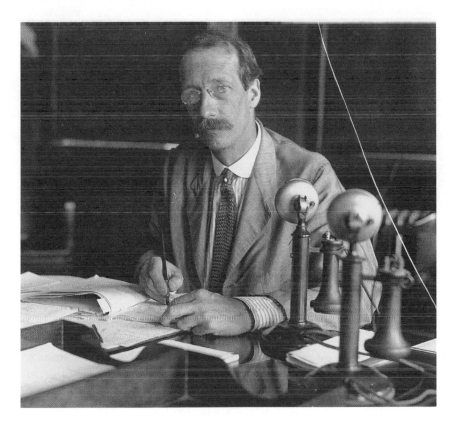

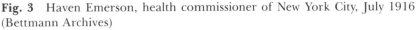

Fig. 3 Haven Emerson, health commissioner of New York City, July 1916
(Bettmann Archives)

in 1923, according to one account, spurred fellow sanitarians to
form what became the American Epidemiological Society.[55] For
some officials, polio work paved the way for a future career.
Wade Hampton Frost, a federal epidemiologist who had studied
polio since 1911, played a prominent role in the professionalization of American epidemiology; later he was chosen the first
professor of epidemiology at the new Johns Hopkins School of
Public Health and Hygiene.[56] But the names of most other polio
fighters in this period have faded now from scientific and medical literature.

The case of polio suggests that tensions between clinicians and laboratory researchers remained unresolved despite professional acceptance of the methods and theories of German research science. Scientists persisted in defining polio as a problem of laboratory-defined etiology rather than investigating its epidemiological or clinical symptoms. They assumed that further study of the characteristics of the polio virus would illuminate the disease's progress in the human body and the community. But the hopes that the laboratory would solve the problem of polio were mostly in vain, and the greatest insights during this period came from observations made in the field and at the bedside.

To most epidemiologists and health officials, fighting polio epidemics was a technical problem. Rather than debate polio's etiological characteristics, workers in the field tried to establish the length of infection, the role of carriers, and the mechanism of transmission. They drew their analyses of insect vectors from Walter Reed's work on yellow fever and mosquitoes and the significance of healthy carriers from Emil Behring's discovery of hidden diphtheria cases. Knowing the shape of an etiological agent played little part for their determining a disease's clinical and epidemiological characteristics.

Epidemics challenged the extent of integrating laboratory techniques in medical practice and lay understanding. The introduction of new tools and techniques was not achieved immediately or smoothly. In the case of polio, the choice of appropriate techniques for diagnosis, therapy, and prevention was negotiated between practitioners and patients, city officials and city dwellers.

Paul Starr has argued that the growth of medical authority in the Progressive era was related to the success of "science in medicine" and the popular recognition of "the inadequacy of unaided and uneducated senses."[57] In this work I argue, however, that the new techniques and technology of scientific medicine were interpreted by both doctor and patient with caution and flexibility. Although members of the public wrote to Simon Flexner and other experts during the 1916 epidemic, they sought more than scientific expertise. Their letters demonstrate their strong sense of the value of empirical reasoning, domestic knowledge, and lay medical skills. Similarly, the germ theory and its ability to explain and control the dirt and disorder of a society were only partially integrated in popular culture. Germs, in lay thought, did not spread randomly; infection depended on the class, ethnicity, and personal habits of individuals. That such assumptions were shared by many officials as well was made strikingly clear during the 1916 polio epidemic.[58]

This study of responses to epidemic polio allows an exploration of changing conceptions of sickness and health through the interactions of medical professionals and the lay public. In the 1900s and 1910s reactions to epidemic polio suggest that doctors and patients largely resisted developing new conceptions of the meaning of dirt. Dirt remained a sign of disease and disorder.[59] During polio epidemics, public health officials linked the disease to dirty streets, unsanitary food, and immigrant children. The fear of dirt was not, however, universally applied; Americans born in the 1920s and 1930s remember associating swimming pools with polio infection. But in the 1910s officials rarely mentioned swimming pools as a danger in spreading polio; instead most officials urged the public to bathe more frequently either at home or in public baths.[60] But one theme does remain constant: the identification of outsiders defined in class and ethnic terms, as the originators and carriers of a frightening epidemic disease.

CHAPTER TWO

This Dread Spectre: Polio and the New Public Health

In mid-August of 1916 the *New York Times* published a poem dealing with the polio epidemic. In "The Bonds of Motherhood" the writer warned that polio crossed class and ethnic lines and threatened children in urban slums and country resorts:

> Mothers with children far away
> From stifling streets and heat,
> Mothers who ceaseless toil all day,
> Their babies at their feet,
> In common have one prayer, one thought
> "Lord, bless my little child,"—
> The one boon from Heaven sought
> "O Thou, with mercy mild,
> Keep this dread spectre from our door"
> Is the one prayer of rich and poor.[1]

As frightened Americans searched for ways to explain and understand "this dread spectre" they turned to medical experts. Public health officials and private physicians responded with traditional measures of epidemic control—quarantine and sanitation—and also methods of the new scientific medicine. These efforts, the public hoped, would guard the community's health, identify carriers of infection, and prevent the spread of the epidemic. But despite these hopes families none-theless fled the urban centers of the disease for the presumed safety of nearby mountains and shore. Those who could not leave barred their children from public places where infection might spread. The public, calling on health officials to control the epidemic through methods old and new, demonstrated not only a fear of filth and marginal groups but also a faith in science.

To understand how and why communities in the Northeast reacted to the 1916 polio epidemic, we must first acknowledge that the public's reaction expressed the fear that frightening, mysterious epidemics often raise. Of course, epidemics in the United States were not unusual; within the memory of a gen-eration serious epidemics of cholera and yellow fever had threatened American shores, and, despite both sanitary and bacteriological measures, communities still faced regular out-breaks of typhoid and smallpox. That polio epidemics targeted children, too, was not surprising; urban children were subject to constant and sometimes deadly outbreaks of whooping cough, scarlet fever, and measles as well as diarrheal infections.[2]

Nonetheless, the special shape of the response to epidemic polio in the 1910s also reflected critical and specific cultural anxieties and expectations. As both health professionals and members of the public tried to explain and control the epi-demic, their efforts raised several questions: the relations among dirt, poverty, the environment, and disease; the long-standing link between immigrants and epidemics; and the new hope of science. Contemporaries had hoped that the issue of assigning responsibility for an epidemic would be answered simply and objectively through the authority of the new scien-tific medicine and the germ theory of disease, hopes that had been boosted by the successes of bacteriology during the previ-ous twenty years. Instead, polio epidemics in this period high-lighted the ambiguities of the power of science.

In 1916 physicians and the public were aware of changes in medical science and public health. But, as responses to the 1916 epidemic demonstrated, both the public's and the profession's acceptance of the transition from sanitary science to New Public

Health remained incomplete. Nor had Progressive reformers' reliance on science and efficiency resolved the controversial role of the state in issues of social and medical reform: the germ theory continued to be interpreted in an expansive framework in which political demands and cultural prejudices played a dominant role. Indeed, significant tensions remained between the lay public and health officials over the proper role of a health department, particularly in its efforts to prevent the appearance and spread of disease. The New Public Health was a concrete ideal, but, in practice, the strained circumstances of an epidemic made visible its intellectual and institutional cracks.

The public health campaign against epidemic polio in 1916 demonstrated the strength of traditional fears of filth and the link between disease carriers and the alien poor. Middle-class citizens associated the appearance and spread of disease with recent immigrants living in city slums. Physicians, health officials, and some members of the public trusted that the germ theory could offer insight into the cause and nature of disease, but they did not believe that germs spread disease randomly. Disease germs were associated with specific kinds of places and people. Native-born middle-class citizens supported official attempts to close immigrant festivals and to restrict mingling across class lines by banning all children from attending movie theaters and other public places of entertainment. Immigrant parents feared both the restrictions and the disease. Many turned to health officials, and departments were, according to one reporter, beseiged all day by men, women and children, "mostly foreigners," demanding medical service.[3] But as they turned to scientific experts in trying to understand and control the disease among their own families, their responses also reflected resentment of the actions of health officials and the extensive use of official power on the streets.

The official response to these fears was typically expansive. During the epidemic, health officials drew on methods from both the New Public Health and sanitary science: quarantine to calm the public and identify and restrict the movement of likely carriers; sanitation and education to prevent the spread of polio and guard public health; and a campaign against a suspected nonhuman carrier, the fly. Such efforts tended to appease rather than undermine these older fears.

QUARANTINE

Health officials had to deal with families fleeing the urban centers of disease and those staying behind. Officials tried to restrict movement, identify the sick and infected, and calm the public. Initially this work strongly drew on the traditional methods of sanitary science. Health reformers defined safe places as those with clean air and surroundings; the countryside, the newly renovated hospital, the properly cleaned home. Those who continued to engage in behavior termed dirty and dangerous needed to be controlled. In practice, most official quarantine measures sought to regulate the behavior of immigrant families as the most effective way to control the spread of the epidemic.

Charitable organizations regularly sent poor mothers and children out of the city during the summer months. Trips to the mountains and seaside were believed to help them regain health and escape the stultifying urban atmosphere. But in 1916 the threat of spreading polio halted these efforts. The New York Association for the Improvement of the Poor and the Newark Female Charitable Society restricted their annual summer outings and announced in local newspapers that this summer some "tired mothers, undernourished children and sickly babies of the tenements" would be denied "Cool, Restful, Health-Giving" country air.[4] William Harvey Young, an assistant pastor directing a summer Bible school in downtown Manhattan, noted in a letter to his wife that health officials told fresh air organizers "they must not bring people out [of the city] . . . on account of the epidemic. And that means that the mothers will have to remain here, of course. They will be disappointed."[5]

Many community members shared a belief in the health-giving qualities of country air. Young discussed the restrictions with Mrs. Silvano, a local janitor and mother of a nine-month old girl. "She feels so badly that it is not possible to take the children here to the country for fresh air. And it must be a disappointment to some of the mothers who have seen the little fellows come back all browned after two weeks of it in the fields."[6] To some health workers such restrictions meant that the city had become an even more dangerous place for the poor. Angry at the restrictions, a social worker warned that "conditions are dreadful here. . . . We cannot send any of our poor children away, and that means they must stay in the hot, dirty houses in the hot, dirty streets without a change of any kind. I fear there will be as many deaths from that as from the 'disease' as it is called by the poor."[7]

Nor did health officials' assessments of the epidemic's extent calm the public. Reflecting the popular belief, exemplified by the work of charitable associations, that country air was safe and health-giving, families fled the diseased city for mountain resorts and the Atlantic coast. Health officials were torn between encouraging this escape to safer environs and acknowledging that even these distant areas were not free of the disease. Haven Emerson was embarrassed when the New York daily papers reported his warning that the state Health Department had found a number of polio cases in nearby mountain resort towns in the Catskills. Hotel owners and other resort proprietors were outraged that their towns were now tainted with reports of the disease. After acrimonious public debate Emerson withdrew his general warning and admitted that he had really been talking about only four upstate towns. But hotel keepers feared the damage was already done.[8]

In July and August 1916, as the front pages of daily newspapers displayed the growing number of cases and deaths, public panic grew. Well-to-do parents fled the urban centers, particularly New York City, the center of the epidemic. Neighboring communities, fearing that New York City children were infected, pressured public health officials to regulate their movement and identify possible disease carriers. Officials' fervent efforts to enforce a quarantine against traveling carriers were visible and dramatic ways to calm the public, part of a traditional approach in dealing with epidemic disease. In spite of fervent debate over the worth of local and state quarantine,

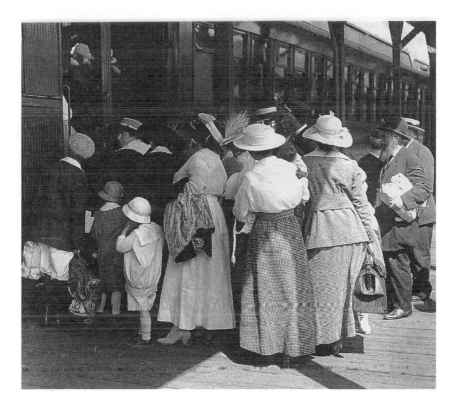

Fig. 4   Women and children flee New York City during 1916 epidemic (Bettmann Archives)

New Jersey, Pennsylvania, Rhode Island, and Connecticut nonetheless established state quarantines. Pennsylvania State Health Commissioner Samuel G. Dixon sent medical inspectors to guard state border entrances and tried to calm the citizens of his commonwealth by blaming the epidemic on New York travelers. "These radical measures," Dixon later reflected, were "demanded by the public, and our want of knowledge forbade our resisting the wish of those whom we represented, and whose health and lives had been entrusted to our care."[9] Faced with this stigma as the center and origin of the epidemic, New York state officials rejected the idea of a state quarantine and left the decision to local boards of health.[10]

Just who was a carrier of polio was not resolved by scientific experts. Bacteriologists could not identify polio carriers with the certainty that they had displayed in the case of Typhoid Mary a few years earlier. Other signs came to stand for polio infection: families from New York City were immediate targets. Many local health boards began to prohibit New York City children from staying or even traveling through their towns. Poughkeepsie, for example, barred any "suspicious person" and announced a two-week quarantine period for all other visitors.[11] Residents of Setauket, Long Island, posted a placard stating:

> "Warning.—We are informed that families from the infected parts of New York City and Brooklyn are offering high prices for rooms and houses here. While we sympathize fully with all who are suffering from this dread disease, infantile paralysis, we certainly should be very careful to whom we extend the hospitality of our village, that the dread disease may not make its appearance here."[12]

In a few cases, public hysteria exacerbated fears of all travelers and strangers. In July, officials in Patterson, New Jersey, announced that until further notice no "nonresidents" would be allowed to stay in that town, no matter where they were from.[13]

New York City officials were quick to respond. By mid-July, although critical of the community "hysteria," Haven Emerson introduced a system of health certificates. His department offered to examine any child traveling outside the city and certify that the child was not infected and had not been staying in an infected neighborhood. These certificates gave communities outside New York City one way to assess whether a child was free of infection. By the end of the epidemic the Health Department had issued 68,000 certificates and refused 348 applicants.[14]

Other city health departments, including Philadelphia and Camden, adopted a similar certificate system, and Hermann Biggs, New York's state health commissioner, helped Emerson extend his certificate system across the state. Federal officials from the U.S. Public Health Service provided their own inspectors and certificates to deal with interstate travelers.[15] Health

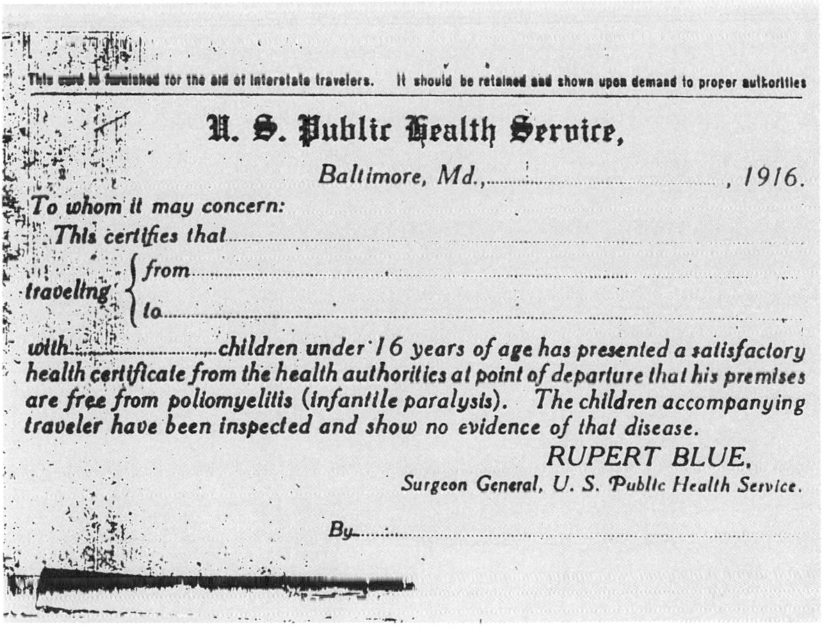

This card is furnished for the aid of interstate travelers. It should be retained and shown upon demand to proper authorities

U. S. Public Health Service,

Baltimore, Md.,.................................., 1916.

To whom it may concern:
This certifies that...
traveling { *from*...
{ *to*...
with...........................*children under 16 years of age has presented a satisfactory
health certificate from the health authorities at point of departure that his premises
are free from poliomyelitis (infantile paralysis). The children accompanying
traveler have been inspected and show no evidence of that disease.*
RUPERT BLUE,
Surgeon General, U. S. Public Health Service.

By..........:..........

Fig. 5 U.S. Public Health Service certificate for children traveling during 1916 epidemic (National Archives)

certificates, an accepted part of public health work, reflected official and popular assumptions of the link between contagion and location.[16] Other health regulations also made explicit the class bias of the urban control of disease. Placards warning of the presence of a polio case (in various languages) were to be hung outside only tenements and dwellings with more than one family; private houses and single family dwellings were considered less dangerous. Significantly, a health certificate from a private physician was not considered sufficient evidence that a child was "free of infection." Certificates had to be signed by health officials.[17] Some practitioners, clearly, were trusted neither to provide accurate diagnoses nor to put the community's good before the convenience of their own patients.

These certificates were, however, unconvincing. New York children were frequently refused entrance to neighboring towns or else threatened with quarantines as long as four weeks. One town in Long Island posted large red signs on the main entrance roads warning travelers that, certificate or no, children would not be allowed to pass through their community.[18]

Private physicians and some health officials admitted that polio was difficult to diagnose, its spread mysteriously unpredictable. A simple clinical inspection could not determine whether a child had the disease. Determining the appropriate length of quarantine was a further problem. Polio experts were not sure exactly how long a child afflicted with polio remained infectious.[19] In any case, polio did not seem to be very contagious, compared to other reportable infectious diseases. In fact, it was rare for more than one child in a family to fall victim to paralysis. Nonetheless, most health officials felt that, when in doubt, they should apply the severest quarantine measures. "The general policy is to look at the disease as closely as we would look at a case of smallpox," Charles F. Bolduan, the director of health education in New York City, told reporters in July. [20]

The use of certificates expanded as the epidemic continued and public panic intensified. Families streamed out of New York City by train, in automobiles, via streetcars, and on private boats. Taxed to their limit, inspectors checking health certificates were on occasion forced to chase fleeing children through unsympathetic crowds. Gradually, however, the specificity of diagnosis diminished. Philadelphia officials were faced with the problem of children from nearby Camden entering the city each day to work. In response to complaints by their employers, the city health chief began to issue twenty-four-hour and then weekly health certificates.[21]

THE LITTLE LEPERS AT HOME

Officials had to deal with families at home as well as those on the move. They urged strict quarantine measures, and the public responded with fear and at times hysteria. In her poem "The Little Lepers" a New York writer exaggerated the implications of quarantine measures:

The city is too full of them, the country is afraid of them;
Turn them from the village and drive them from the town
They must not tarry in the street, they cannot stifle in the
house;
Wherever they may wander, hunt them up and drive them
down . . . [concluding]
Strange ones, familiar ones, keep them from the loved
ones!
Your child and my child had better play apart,
Until there comes an ending to this terror-stricken hour,
When we turn away from children with horror in the
heart![22]

There was less concern with institutional quarantine, for the epidemic occurred during the summer when the school year in most communities had ended. Orphanages and children's homes unable to discharge their inmates barred all visitors and began cleanliness campaigns. Children's summer camps either abandoned their sites or isolated themselves from parents and other children. A boys' camp in Fort Hamilton, for example, quarantined itself and accepted no new boys.[23] Families that did not send their sick children to a hospital were placarded by the health department. A typical sign, in red on white paper, read:

> Board of Health of Newark, New Jersey. Keep Out. This house contains a case of infantile paralysis. Any person violating the isolation and quarantine rules and regulations of the board, or who willfully removes, defaces or obstructs this card without authority is liable to a fine of $50.[24]

As the epidemic stretched into August, health officials convinced legislators to extend the emergency powers of city and state health departments. In Pennsylvania Dixon gave full police power to all state health inspectors to make arrests without warrants of families suspected of hiding an infected child.[25]

Official action also stressed the danger of congregating children. After conferring with his medical advisors and head of the city's education department Haven Emerson decided to postpone opening the city's public schools. The decision occasioned much debate, although finally most schools opened only two weeks later than usual. Concerned college administrators responded by also postponing their usual openings. Some colleges also temporarily banned students who had stayed in "infected districts" over the summer.[26] Public health officials in Philadelphia barred churches and Sunday schools from accepting children under sixteen during the epidemic.[27] Whether the results of official action or public fear, church attendance did decline. William Young, the New York pastor, noted that his Bible school class "did not have a very large crowd, due again to the suspicion of danger of disease, I take it."[28]

To the consternation of the public, during debates over the extension of health official power, polio experts were seen to disagree. In New Jersey the Newark Health Department conducted a running public battle with the city's school superintendent who did not believe that closing school playgrounds during the summer months benefited either mothers or children. After a meeting in which twenty-six doctors divided evenly on the question, and the board of education argued in favor of the safety of a clean, medically supervised school, a local reporter commented that "it would have been difficult to find a better example of the divided opinion[s] of medical men and the laity as to the proper methods for checking the disease spread than that of last night."[29]

One safe place, according to health officials, was the city hospital. The quarantine conditions imposed by the New York City health department during the 1916 epidemic were so strict that many parents were forced to send their sick children to a hospital. Requirements for domestic quarantine included a private toilet for the patient, separate dining facilities, and a private nurse.[30] No tenement dweller could have complied. Yet, for many families, hospitals, particularly those run by the city, retained their traditional reputation as dark places for the destitute and dying.[31]

Emerson had anticipated difficulties in convincing families to obey quarantine rules. He fervently praised his department's contagious disease hospitals, assuring the public that they were not "what are commonly feared as pest houses." Their polio wards were "all open, airy, sunny, cheerful rooms, where children not only receive the best of care and attention, but where they have the advantages of absolutely sanitary and healthful surroundings not possible in many homes." This comparison with the dark, crowded, and unsanitary homes of poor children of the city was a constant theme. Emerson reminded parents that by agreeing to have their child taken to a hospital they could also "lessen the chances of their children catching the disease by proper precautions."[32] Similarly, the Philadelphia Department of Health noted that only one-quarter as many New York children had died in hospitals as at home, and it urged parents to "give your child the benefit of the greater chances of recovery and permit it to be sent to the City Hospital."[33]

But many poor families remained unwilling to have their children go to a public hospital. One mother warned a doctor that if he claimed her child had "that disease" and reported her to the Health Department she and her child would be gone by the next morning.[34] In resisting official attempts to send afflicted children to local hospitals, parents were reaffirming a long-standing popular fear that hospitals were a source of infection. A Newark health inspector was hit by a brick thrown by angry Italian "excited women" protesting the removal of a child to the city's isolation hospital.[35] And after the health officer of Oyster Bay, Long Island, suggested that children with polio from outside the local area be brought to the Glen Cove isolation hospital, he received a death threat and a warning that the hospital would be burned down.[36]

Outside major urban centers the question of where to house polio victims quickly divided many communities. The isolation wards of those private hospitals that agreed to accept polio cases were soon filled.[37] Quarantine measures became sources of conflict as parents refused to accede to health officials' demands. Members of the public were warned of the dangers of the city but were prohibited from leaving. Parents, particularly recent immigrants, feared that sick children were mistakenly diagnosed, and did not accept health officials' designation. A Brooklyn woman protested that her child, a "suspicious case," should not be taken to the city's Kingston Avenue Hospital, on the grounds that he did not have the disease but would catch it from other children there. In a compromise measure, the Health Department took the child but placed him in quarters separate from those occupied by positive cases.[38]

This health campaign reinforced many immigrant families' deep fears of the mysterious disease. There had been few previous polio outbreaks in Europe or the United States, and the unfamiliar disease was frightening. Parents locked their children in stuffy rooms and boarded up windows to block possibly infected air.[39] Health workers found it difficult to convince immigrant parents of the benefits of fresh air and outdoor play when faced with polio's high death rate. "I do not wonder they are afraid," reflected a New York social worker. "I went to see one family about 4 P.M. Friday. The baby was not well and the doctor was coming. When I returned Monday morning there were three little hearses before the door, all her children had been swept away in that short time. The mothers are hiding their children rather than give them up."[40]

The fear of spreading the disease through the indiscriminate mingling of children led officials to engage in unusually restrictive measures. Local New Jersey officials were particularly active, and the state's Department of Health decided not to interfere, although one newspaper editor warned that public feelings were "wrought up to a high pitch."[41] In mid-July, for the first time in Newark's history, the city had a childless circus, and a few days later the Harry Lukens Wild Animal Show, which had pitched its tent in downtown Newark, was ordered to leave without giving a single performance.[42] The city's superintendent of schools postponed a summer spelling bee. Patterson officials closed Sunday schools and barred a Boy Scouts' matinee at the local movie house.[43]

Immigrant neighborhoods were special targets for official action. Officials monitored immigrant festivals, working-class block parties, and public playgrounds. The New York City Health Department canceled the annual three-day celebration of the Italian feast day of Our Lady of Mount Carmel. When inspecting the recreational center at Starr Garden, a city settlement house, Philadelphia officials examined children whose appearance suggested "unsanitary home conditions."[44] The class bias of this campaign was particularly evident. Philadelphia official Wilmer Krusen, for example, imposed a quarantine ban on neighborhood street carnivals and parties, but he agreed to issue permits for lawn fetes, if they were roped off and conducted under police supervision to ensure that no children under sixteen attended. Perhaps health officials felt it was impossible to control working-class festivals but hoped middle-class families might be more willing to cooperate.[45]

As the epidemic wore on, quarantine measures also increasingly conflicted with economic activity. During August, the mayor of Asbury Park, New Jersey, conducted a running battle with the town's medical officer, who had suggested canceling the nationally renowned Asbury Park Baby Parade, which had, so one newspaper claimed, made the town's reputation and signaled the best "revenue producing day" for the town's stores, hotels, and amusement places.[46] By mid-August the mayor said that he was "sick of the whole business" and did not care if the parade was held or not.[47] The parade was finally canceled but only after federal officials stepped in and reminded the mayor and protesting businessmen that, profits aside, a mass assembly of babies would not only be an ideal environment for spreading polio, but, if cases of polio appeared, bad publicity for the town as well.[48]

Organizers of other summer entertainments also suffered. In July Emerson instructed all motion picture exhibitors in New York City to bar children under sixteen from entering theaters and threatened reluctant managers with the loss of their licenses. At first exhibitors, happy to assist the city's health department, offered their screens to publicize polio prevention rules.[49] But as the epidemic stretched into the summer they became less enthusiastic and complained about losing receipts during their busiest season. The prohibition hurt children of all classes, they pointed out. An officer of the Motion Picture Exhibitors League told reporters that he believed the ban would particularly hurt nickel-and-dime outdoor theaters such as the Nickelodeons and Airdromes and that dozens of theaters in the

Lower East Side and Brooklyn would be forced to close.[50] Owners of other entertainment enterprises for children also became
upset as parents, heeding health department warnings, kept
their families away. Coney Island and Brighton Beach lost most
of their regular summer crowds, and Atlantic City entrepreneurs conducted an extensive publicity campaign to convince
visitors of the safety of the New Jersey shore.[51]

CLEANLINESS

Perhaps the only business interests that benefited during the
epidemic as the result of health officials' actions were enterpris-
ing manufacturers of hygienic products. Advertisers expanded
on health department warnings about the importance of domestic hygiene by offering products to disinfect the nose and
mouth. "Cleanliness in the home is the best preventive of this
dread disease," promised one advertiser, and " 'Crexol' is the
best of all disinfectants for cleaning."[52] Similarly, Rexall's tooth-
paste would "preserve the teeth [and] strengthen the gums" as
it removed "dangerous germs which infect the mouth and
throat."[53]

Rumors that physicians were bringing infection home to their
families also appeared in these advertisements. After four-year-
old Elizabeth Chalmers died of the disease, her father, Thomas
C. Chalmers, head of the visiting staff of the Queens Borough
Hospital for Contagious Diseases, announced that he did not
believe his work with polio patients was responsible for the
death of his daughter.[54] But at least one advertiser retold the
story of a physician whose daughter had become infected, possibly by "parasites or germs carried home by her father who has
been attending several cases of this disease." Such a case could
have been prevented by the use of Fitzgerald's Hair Soap which
"kills contagious disease-carrying parasites, and also all nits and
fleas and germs."[55]

During the 1916 epidemic, city health departments conducted extensive cleanup campaigns focused on both public

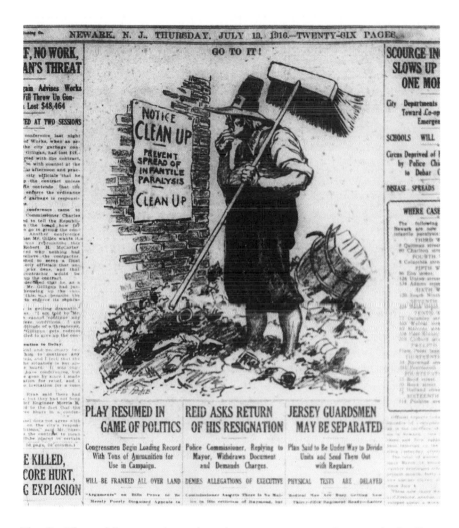

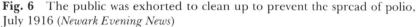

Fig. 6 The public was exhorted to clean up to prevent the spread of polio, July 1916 (*Newark Evening News*)

and private hygiene. In this time of public panic, despite their emulation of the work of New Public Health proponent Charles Chapin, health officials tried to assuage public fear by emphasizing their fight against both dirt and germs. Even progressive departments reverted to methods that were part of an older sanitary tradition. Although New York City, for example, had formally abolished its system of public fumigation and disinfection a year earlier, old public health traditions reasserted themselves during the 1916 epidemic as city officials flushed streets with chloride of lime, removed garbage, ashes, and refuse from congested districts, arrested householders and storekeepers who broke sanitary regulations, and forced tenants to clean up halls, cellars, and yards.[56]

At first glance, this emphasis on sanitation simply reflected attempts to combine environmental with individual health reform. These efforts were designed to inspire members of the public to clean their homes and persons. In theory, such cleanup campaigns were targeted at everyone: the immigrant and native-born, tenement and suburban dweller, parents and children. Such a broad approach, in which each individual had equal responsibility in guarding the public health, was clearly part of the New Public Health. The focus on all homes, including those of the middle class, appeared justified by polio's appearance in both suburbs and slums.

But in practice some groups were seen as more responsible than others. Officials, seeing poor and immigrant families as dirty and germ-ridden carriers of the disease, directed their primary efforts toward these unfortunate groups. These measures mirrored the fears of middle-class urbanites, suggesting that the epidemic was spreading in one direction: from the tenements to the suburbs. The emphasis on sanitation, then, offered both the public and the medical profession a way to define and explain the epidemic. Polio conceived as a dirt disease could resolve questions of responsibility for the spread of polio; sanitation became a means of protection and prediction. This traditional emphasis also suggested that the conceptual implications of the germ theory were neither fully accepted nor understood. Germs might be everywhere, but public health work tended to divide cases into guilty carriers and innocent victims.

The cleanup campaign also continued nineteenth-century nativist elements in public health work. By the early decades of this century it had become commonplace to blame immigrants for heightened urban public health problems. To native-born Americans, the East European groups that had been arriving in northeastern cities since the 1880s seemed especially alien. By this time, native-born Americans no longer blamed epidemics on the Irish and Germans, immigrants of a previous generation. Indeed, Irish and German families had become so accepted a part of the urban American landscape that some officials now categorized their children with those of native-born families. Epidemiological studies assumed that such families, unlike most recent Italian, Polish, and Russian immigrants, shared similar living conditions and standards of domestic hygiene.[57]

Anti-polio sanitary campaigns centered on specific districts where Eastern European immigrant families lived. The slums of South Philadelphia and the Lower East Side of Manhattan were called, almost interchangeably, "congested" and "infected."[58] This work mixed education with cleanliness; officials removed garbage and other filth from the streets of specific districts as they urged residents to improve their own domestic hygiene. In New York City, Philadelphia, and Newark, tenement districts were plastered with health department pamphlets and placards in Italian, Yiddish, and Slavic, all warning immigrant mothers of the dangers of the disease and unsanitary living.[59] Although recent immigrant groups lived mostly in northeastern cities, a few observers feared that infected immigrants could spread the disease nationally. In Washington, during a congressional debate on the epidemic, Georgia representative William Schley Howard threatened to oppose legislation involving the use of Ellis Island as a holding center for polio patients, on the grounds that "immigrants would carry the disease to children all over the country."[60]

The idea that overcrowding, poverty, and sanitary ignorance bred disease was firmly incorporated in official actions against epidemic polio. But even cursory studies tracing the spread of polio cases pointed to inconsistencies in this view. Andrew

Cairns, a Philadelphia health officer, noted that there were few polio cases in the city's "congested" lower wards compared to the neighborhoods north of the city "where new houses and little congestion are generally factors in keeping down death and disease rate[s] from other forms of illness."[61] These neighborhoods had the highest numbers of polio cases reported, but epidemiologists discovered later that "congested districts" had lower rates of polio than suburban and rural districts in the Greater New York area. A Pennsylvania county medical inspector was similarly puzzled by the spread of the epidemic in Chester County, a region "populated by wealthy, seclusive, and sanitary homes; part of it by the opposite—dirty, careless and thoughtless families; and . . . there seemed to be no difference between the character of the homes as to the fruits of the disease."[62]

Cases that appeared in the fashionable New York City's Upper East Side and Philadelphia's Main Line made front page news. Readers were spared few details, for example, of the illness and death of newly married twenty-five-year-old Mrs. Catherine Sefton Page, daughter-in-law of Walter Hines Page, the American ambassador to France. Her death, according to the editor of the *New York Times,* "shocked the community" for "it has shown strikingly how subtle and uncontrolled are the ravages of the strange epidemic which still baffles the physicians, [and] has already destroyed so many young lives." Catherine Page, reporters noted, lived in surroundings "that were considered ideal and decidedly inimical to the existence of paralysis germs, yet she contracted the plague."[63] In Philadelphia Charles B. Shakespeare, a "young society man," was the city's first adult victim in 1916. On the front page of the *Evening Bulletin* a reporter remarked that "considerable agitation ensued in the exclusive districts along the Main Line when the news became current that infantile paralysis had penetrated to that exclusive section where immunity should seem certain if it were possible at all."[64]

Officials attempted to distinguish safe from unsafe neighborhoods and to present middle-class polio victims as anomalous. But defining and targeting dangerous districts did not confine the spread of the epidemic. In fact, such efforts reinforced the

dangerous nature of the public urban sphere.[65] Nor did it allay
suburbanites' continuing fear of infection crossing class boundaries into the private sphere. Middle-class parents worried that,
although their private homes were far from the "infected" tenement districts, their children could be endangered by public
interaction with poor immigrant children. Children might play
together in the same playground and sandpile, share a streetcar
seat, drink from the same soda fountain glass, or use the same
public library book, toy, or piece of clothing that had been returned to a store. Polio could endanger middle-class families
through their public interaction with families from "infected"
districts.[66]

Health officials responded to these fears by closing playgrounds, disinfecting sandpiles, and enforcing the strict cleanliness of soda fountain services. Librarians closed children's
reading rooms; streetcars and public telephones were disinfected nightly by companies fearful of losing customers.[67] After
three children who had played in a local park were reported
sick, Philadelphia health officials ordered the Board of Recreation to disinfect the playground. Officials not only cleaned
public spaces but also, in some cases, turned them into medical
centers. In Philadelphia, as part of the citywide campaign to
supervise children, many playgrounds were converted into
open-air clinics. By early August 23 recreation centers and 138
school playgrounds were reopened as health centers, staffed
with nurses, sanitary inspectors, and members of local medical
societies, including the Homeopathic Medical Club and the
Philadelphia Physicians' Motor Club.[68] But many families, un-
convinced that these measures were sufficient, continued to
flee the cities during July and August.[69]

Blaming the spread of the disease on the irresponsible sanitary behavior of immigrants could help explain the appearance
of polio among wealthy families. Germs carried by immigrants,
some feared, could enter suburban houses and bring infection
and death. In one case, an eminent physician used this fear to
refute an argument about doctors carrying polio out of the
hospital and into their own homes and communities. One of his
children had died of the disease, but, the father explained, it

was not the result of his work with polio patients. He always washed his hands thoroughly and changed immediately into street clothes when he came home. Nor was his family allowed to enter his medical office. No, the carrier of the fatal disease into his home was his children's Polish nurse who had thoughtlessly visited her sister's family where there was an infected child, a family where doubtless proper sanitation was neither observed nor understood. Haven Emerson told this story to a group of health officials during a national conference on polio. He commented that the nurse "with her habits, coming from an infected child, appeared to us and to the doctor who lost the child as the more probable carrier."[70] The notion of polio carriers as selective transmitters of the polio germ helped reinforce the official picture of the epidemic radiating out from immigrant slums and endangering middle-class homes.

EDUCATION

Health officials tried not only to ameliorate social conditions but also to inspire individuals to change their behavior and thought. Anti-polio campaigns, however, suffered from a lack of specific preventive measures. Scientists had suggested that this disease, although imperfectly understood, could be controlled by attention to personal and domestic hygiene. In July 1916 polio expert Simon Flexner told a large audience at the prestigious New York Academy of Medicine that his experimental work at the Rockefeller Institute had shown that polio was spread mainly by kissing, coughing, and sneezing.[71] Other experts also emphasized that personal contact could be dangerous.[72] When polio cases did appear in unlikely locations, health officials and private physicians tried to explain them by blaming parents' hygienic carelessness and ignorance. "A large majority of the cases," argued the editor of the New York Times, "have been found in families where such instruction is needed."[73]

Teaching the public about the danger of germ-laden secretions was an integral part of the New Public Health. Health education was to be, Chapin and other promoters stressed, the

If a case of infantile paralysis occurs in your home your doctor must at once notify the Department of Health. An inspector will be sent to investigate. He will paste a sign on the door of your house and apartment warning all people not to enter. This sign must not be removed except by some one sent by the Department of Health. The inspector and nurse will tell you just what to do to protect yourself and the others in the family.

Should you want any further information write or telephone to the

DEPARTMENT OF HEALTH

139 CENTRE STREET, NEW YORK

Telephone 6280 Franklin

[The other side of this leaflet bore the following:]

INFANTILE PARALYSIS IS DANGEROUS!

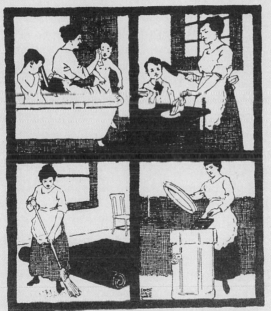

CLEAN UP AND KEEP CLEAN!

KEEP your children clean. Bathe them frequently. See that they keep their hands particularly clean. Be sure that each child has its own clean handkerchief.

Keep your house unusually clean. Don't allow a fly in it. Keep your garbage bucket clean and tightly covered.

Have a general house-cleaning. Throw away all useless knick-knacks and rubbish. Use soap and water generously, and let nature kill the germs with sunshine and fresh air.

Fig. 7 Part of health leaflet issued by New York City Department of Health during 1916 epidemic (Haven Emerson, *A Monograph on The Epidemic of Poliomyelitis [Infantile Paralysis] in New York City in 1916. Based on the Official Reports of the Bureaus of the Department of Health* [New York: Department of Health, 1917])

strong arm of this new approach to public health work, and by the 1910s it had become an important part of many city health departments' mission. In 1915 New York City had established a separate Bureau of Public Health Education, with its own director and staff. Using a variety of media—leaflets, talks to school children and physicians, exhibits, slides and motion pictures, and 126 health bulletins in 1916 alone, many of them published and discussed in the local press—the Bureau conducted campaigns about the dangers of sneezing, mosquitoes, and venereal disease quackery. In mid-July the Bureau screened the Rockefeller Institute film *Fighting Infantile Paralysis* at special matinee sessions for mothers in infected districts.[74]

Health education appealed to officials, who tried to resolve the troubling problems of responsibility for this disease. Officials sought to have mothers and housekeepers assume the critical role of guarding their homes from dirt and disease. Families in "infected" districts were believed to have ignored the laws of sanitary science and the expertise of medical practitioners.

Officials wanted to play the role of enlightened landlords: providing a sanitary environment and dealing with the behavior of urban tenants. After touring the Brooklyn neighborhood where the first polio cases had been reported, Emerson announced that his department would be strictly enforcing the city's tenement regulations, particularly regarding garbage piles and unscreened windows.[75] The Philadelphia Housing Association distributed thousands of leaflets to tenants; the publications informed them of their "sanitation rights" but added that "sickness and death from contagious diseases are unnecessary and that thousands of cases need not occur if proper attention is taken in cleanliness and sanitation."[76] Thus, families held the responsibility for health in their own hands. The emphasis on the importance of domestic hygiene promised ordinary citizens a sense of possible control and protection, a feeling reinforced by advertisers of sanitary products who combined threats of public disorder with promises of safety through individual control. Just as Emerson directed the Street Cleaning Department of New York City to sprinkle all "infected" streets with water and flush them at night, so, on a more intimate scale, Emerson asked New

York housewives to do the same and use tea leaves when sweeping to ensure that they collected as much dangerous dust as possible.[77]

Officials tried to identify the sick, the unclean, the irresponsible, and the ignorant and to teach them the rules of sanitation. Rather than play down the extent of epidemics as his predecessors had done, Haven Emerson deliberately chose not to hide the number of polio cases from the public. He used the media to inform the public of cases, deaths, and health guidelines, and every day newspapers printed addresses and gave a running total. In Philadelphia and Newark city officials, adopting similar policies, urged members of the public to look for symptoms of disease and to contact their private physician or board of health.

Notices in the daily papers, health pamphlets, and slides at movie theaters stressed that strict sanitary care could protect a home and child from the disease. Parents were warned particularly to guard the behavior of their children. One Newark official told parents to avoid caressing or kissing children, to forbid children from buying fruit or other exposed foods from street vendors, and to keep them from exchanging toys, marbles, candy, or chewing gum.[78] Newark kindergarten teachers were warned not to teach their students games or dances that required personal contact.[79] One Philadelphia newspaper editor reminded his readers that most infant mortality was avoidable, a result mainly from the "reckless disregard of accepted measures of precaution and care." A wise parent would heed the rules from official bulletins.[80] Broad environmental issues continued to be important in public health efforts, but the "environment" was increasingly limited to the wash basin, the toilet, and the garbage can.

Although health officials stressed that poor personal hygiene left children vulnerable to the disease, this argument was not, however, supported by contemporary epidemiological reports. Prominent scientists acknowledged that the strong and affluent were victims as frequently as the weak. "In all homes where polio exists," a Philadelphia paper reported, "children have been declared well nourished and cared for."[81] "Vigorous

health seems to be no protection against the disease," Simon
Flexner commented in a New York newspaper.[82] Philadelphia's
Wilmer Krusen acknowledged that the disease "comes where
we least look for it, and under conditions we never think of.
There is no explanation, geographically, that [we] can give."[83]
Despite such statements, the messages of health education re-
mained unaltered.

Health education was not always welcomed by its recipients.
Public health nurses and social workers, who entered the homes
of the immigrant poor, sought to transform their lives through
education and the aid of city services. Some families to whom
this education campaign was directed, however, resisted the
assistance. In late July a nurse employed at a Brooklyn baby
health station told police that she had received a "Black Hand"
letter threatening her if she continued to report unsanitary
conditions and suspicious polio cases among local Italian families: "If you report any more of our babies to the Board of
Health we will kill you and nobody will know what happened to
you. Keep off our streets and don't report our homes and we
will do you no harm." According to one newspaper, the letter
was written in blood.[84]

As a result, in dealing with working-class families, some of
these efforts at inspection and education shifted into enforcement. In mid-August, for example, nurses supplied by several
New York charity organizations began investigations of tenement families in order to discover what they believed were numerous hidden polio cases.[85] The nurses used the opportunity
to report any families who might be charity cases, as well as
those who had violated food laws, illegally occupied premises,
and improperly cleaned streets, cellars, and yards. During their
inspections nurses also tried to educate these families, warning
parents against bad hygienic habits such as lack of bathing,
neglect of toilets, poor water supply (many families still used
wells), improper feeding of children, food exposed to heat and
insects, and other practices that could lead to the spread of
disease. But their efforts had limited effect. Any changes tenement families undertook, the nurses observed, were largely due
to the "fear of authority and the force of the department and

not to voluntary action on their parts."[86] Haven Emerson was forced to supplement the authority of his department with the cooperation of city magistrates who enthusiastically fined street vendors and housewives caught with food exposed to flies, uncovered garbage, and other public health violations believed to promote the spread of the epidemic. One magistrate warned that "if you won't cooperate willingly the city will make you do so."[87]

Social workers, similarly, were forced to call on the regulatory powers of health departments when their efforts at persuasion failed. In a letter reprinted in a New York newspaper, social worker Monica Moore told the head of her hospital's social service committee that "in one house I went into the only window was not only shut, but the cracks were stuffed with rags, so that the 'disease' could not come in. You can imagine what the dark, dirty room was like; the babies had no clothes on, and were so wet and hot that they looked as if they had been dipped in oil, and the flies were sticking all over them." Torn between her role as public official and sharing her clients' fear of the unknown disease entering homes without control, Moore continued: "I had to tell the mother I would get the Board of Health after her to make her open the window, and now if any of the children do get infantile paralysis she will feel that I killed them."[88]

Efforts at sanitary regulation became even less popular as the public realized that these mostly nonspecific methods reflected the limited understanding of the disease. Officials admitted, when challenged by both physicians and citizens, that sanitary measures were intended to be educational and only broadly effective. They defended them as a way to build up community resistance, just as personal hygiene was believed to reinforce individual resistance against disease, "creating a general condition of healthfulness and precaution" that would allow the community "to secure immunity from the immediate particular menace."[89] Philadelphia officials reminded the public that "fresh air, sunshine and good food are excellent preventive remedies, for these increase the individual resistance and lessen the susceptibility to infectious disease."[90]

Former allies of health officials, moreover, began to express their resentment. City ministers grew increasingly unhappy about health department bans on Sunday schools. Reverend J. Garland Hamner, the pastor of a Newark church, accused health authorities of exaggerating and creating panic and ignored the ban. There had been more suicides in the past four months in New York City than deaths from infantile paralysis, he claimed, and the danger of infection was in not the clean, light airy classrooms of Sunday schools but trolley cars where passengers from the poorer sections of the city traveled in close contact with those from the suburbs.[91]

Some health officials recognized that their colleagues were engaging in a shotgun approach to the problem of epidemic polio by recommending "every known epidemiological remedy in the hope that one may hit the mark." Still, the "public will select the remedy which suits their fancy," reflected the editor of the *American Journal of Public Health*.[92] New York's anti-polio campaign, he warned, had returned to the "old filth theory of disease," although he had hoped that "this leaf in the history of sanitation" would "never be turned back." Health officials, he argued, should base their work on knowledge, not guesswork. Even in typhoid fever and cholera, a general campaign of cleanliness "usually misses the mark." "A shot-gun policy in public health work is as absurd and useless as an old time shot-gun prescription in therapeutics."[93] Some citizens, however, suggested that sanitation might improve the public health even if it did not halt the spread of polio. In a letter to a daily paper, one Philadelphian pointed out: "The preventative suggestions issued by the health authorities are the sum-total of recognized sanitary and dietetic rules that have no special bearing on [polio] . . . a sort of shotgun effort which is altogether commendable and which will have the effect of improving public health, even if it does not stay infantile paralysis."[94]

These attempts at enforcement, however, illustrate the failure of the New Public Health to allow health officials to transform their role from sanitary regulators to scientific guides and educators. Their efforts at quarantine and sanitation during the 1916 epidemic demonstrated the still contradictory goals of public health work, like Progressive reform in general, which used the state as a benign regulator to monitor the behavior of all groups in society. In theory, as individuals changed their behavior, such regulation would no longer be necessary. But, in practice, public health campaigns were not directed equally at all groups in society. Urban slums and their immigrant tenants were the primary targets of anti-polio campaigns, even when, officials acknowledged, polio victims were also found among native-born, clean, suburban families.

Swat the Fly

> Don't let your children go to parties, picnics or outings.
> Don't let your children play with any children who have sickness at home.
> If your child is sick, send for your doctor at once or send word to the Board of Health.
> A watched child is a safe child.
> Swat the fly.[95]

New York City motion picture screens displayed this notice during the height of the 1916 epidemic. As well as broad warnings about the importance of domestic hygiene, such notices suggested one specific way to protect children from epidemic polio and prevent the spread of the disease: swatting flies. Anti-fly campaigns soon appeared in other cities: in Philadelphia the phrase on everyone's lips was "screen the baby."[96]

The notion that flies spread polio gained popularity for a number of reasons. It intensified a popular association of dirt with disease; it enabled public health officials to develop a specific approach to anti-polio work; and it provided a focus for researching the way epidemic polio spread in a scientific, laboratory-oriented context. Furthermore, anti-fly campaigns facilitated the transformation in public health theory and practice from nineteenth-century sanitary science to the New Public Health. These campaigns offered ways to resolve specific problems of polio's confusing epidemiology. At the same time this approach, beyond its practical appeal, integrated broader critiques about ways to explain the spread of the disease and resolve the thorny questions of responsibility.

Indeed, the emphasis on fly control during the most devastating months of the 1916 epidemic may have helped officials, physicians, and the public to bring the epidemic psychologically "down to size" by offering a visible and manageable target. Health officials tried to convince the public that the disease, even as it spread to "safe" districts, was just another controllable public health problem. Thus, Pennsylvania Health Commissioner Samuel Dixon argued that "the positive identification of a food or insect carrier would constitute one of the biggest boons medical science could offer at this time, not only as a means of strengthening the lines of prevention and protection, but as affording mental relief to many thousands of worried parents whose fears now cause them to see avenues of infection on all sides."[97]

Flies were not the only agent blamed for spreading epidemic polio. Dust, a familiar disease carrier, was also implicated. In 1912, the New York State Department of Health promoted a health exhibit that included "photographs of [an animal] spinal cord of poliomyelitis produced by injection of dust of room occupied by a [human] case of poliomyelitis."[98] A federal epidemiologist investigating a polio epidemic in 1911 sent "sweepings of dust from rooms occupied by patients suffering from poliomyelitis" to be tested by researchers at the Hygienic Laboratory in Washington; the results were inconclusive.[99] The idea that inanimate objects (fomites) could spread disease was also still popular, despite Charles V. Chapin's fervent attack on the fear of fomites as antithetical to the germ theory. Pastor William Young worried that the letters he was writing to his wife during the 1916 epidemic might endanger their three-month-old son. "So far as being afraid of the letters I send to you is concerned," he reflected, "I do not think you need have any fear. I write when my fingers have been washed so that the paper will not be contaminated by them." Nonetheless, he warned that "it might be well not to let him have them, and might do to wash your own hands when they have been read.

But that is carrying caution a good way, and I do not think there is enough danger to warrant it."[100] In New York City any book returned to a public library from an infected house was burned; in New Jersey, guards refused to allow any travelers from New York carrying rags or paper to enter the state.[101] The fear of "infected" books and toys lingered to become part of the 1922 children's classic story *The Velveteen Rabbit*.[102]

Domestic pets were also feared as carriers. Physicians had often urged that sickly animals be killed in times of epidemic, and numerous epidemiologists had noted polio cases where children had played with a pet that subsequently developed signs of paralysis. During the 1916 epidemic Commissioner Hermann Biggs warned all physicians in New York State that domestic animals must be strictly prohibited from the sick room. Philadelphia officials banned dogs and cats from school playgrounds.[103] The public responded fervently to these warnings. New York veterinarians reported that people were killing pets and strays, and the New York Society for the Prevention of Cruelty to Animals rounded up dogs and cats abandoned by fearful owners and destroyed three or four hundred a day.[104] In one extreme case, a woman was reported to have been refused admission to three Connecticut towns because, although she had no child, she was traveling with her cat.[105]

But the idea that the polio virus was being spread by insects was especially popular. The link between insects and epidemic disease reflected, after all, the direction of modern science. The discoveries of the role played by mosquitoes in spreading malaria and yellow fever had been publicized widely, and their proponents Ronald Ross and Walter Reed won international scientific and popular accolades. Some physicians had begun to integrate medical entomology into their practices. A doctor who did "not know the habits of the housefly, the flea, the cockroach, the mosquito, the body louse, and numerous other disease-carrying insects," one man remarked, would be helpless in diagnosing disease, and "it would be quite unsafe to allow him to practice in our families."[106]

By the 1900s medical entomology had become an important part of New Public Health work. Insects offered a way to resolve

the ambiguities of the germ theory in relation to early twentieth-
century public health practice. Among the lay public, germs, the
new invisible agents of disease, were often intermingled with the
filth theory of disease. In July 1916 advertisers of Lysol disinfectant warned the public of the combined dangers of germs, dirt
and ignorance:

> The Invisible Menace
> Because germs are invisible their malignancy is increased a
> million fold.
> No one would hesitate an instant to defend a child attacked
> by a mad dog, yet there are thousands who, even in times
> of epidemic, neglect the gravely important duty of making
> their homes germ proof.
> There still exist thousands who refuse to believe in germs
> because they cannot see them. That is why *there are*
> epidemics.
> It is the duty of every intelligent person to offset as far as
> possible the baleful activity of the ignorant.[107]

The strength of older concepts from sanitary science was
clearly reflected in public health work during the summer of
1916. Health officials as well as the public associated disease
with dirt. As most household insects were clearly signs of unsanitary living conditions, by emphasizing their dangers health officials and physicians could provide the public with practical ways
to attack filth and at the same time focus on specific etiological
agents of disease. The theory that polio was spread by insects
combined older ideas about filth with newer ones about germs
and insect vectors.[108]

The housefly was an especially popular target. The early decades of this century saw the publication of dozens of books and
pamphlets warning the public about the dangers of flies. Proponents drew on work by Walter Reed who had suggested that flies
were a significant factor in spreading typhoid fever in army
camps during the Spanish-American War. A widely quoted study
published in the *Journal of the American Medical Association* by
physician-reformer Alice Hamilton linked flies to a 1902 typhoid

epidemic in Chicago; this influenced officials, as did the efforts of L. O. Howard, head of the federal Bureau of Entomology from 1894 to 1927. He established anti-fly work firmly in standard public health practice through his text *The House Fly: Disease Carrier* (1911). A fervent anti-fly campaigner, Howard argued that the fly could not only carry the germs of enteric disorders such as typhoid fever and dysentery but was also linked to the spread of anthrax, cholera, tuberculosis, and smallpox.[109]

Since the early 1910s flies had been associated with epidemic polio. The examples of yellow fever and malaria, whose previously confusing epidemiologies were clarified when the role of the insect carrier was explicated, promised equal hope for this mysterious disease. Furthermore, the model of medical entomology suggested that perhaps the polio virus entered the body through an insect bite. Although some researchers favored other biting insects such as the bedbug, the biting stable fly proved the most popular agent. Influential studies by Philip Sheppard, an officer of the Massachusetts State Board of Health, and Charles Brues, a Harvard entomologist, found polio could be transmitted from a patient's sick room through stable flies to laboratory monkeys who subsequently developed the disease.[110]

Such was the popularity of this work linking polio and flies that one historian of polio later complained that scientists' interest in the fly overshadowed more insightful work on the appearance of the polio virus in asymptomatic cases.[111] In 1912, at the Fifteenth International Congress on Hygiene and Demography in Washington, D.C., Milton J. Rosenau, a Massachusetts state health officer, presented work that he believed established the critical role of stable flies in spreading epidemic polio. Rosenau had exposed twelve monkeys to "infected" stable flies, and six had developed symptoms of the disease.[112] The delegates' enthusiasm for Rosenau's work contrasted sharply with their lukewarm reception to the more cautious experimental studies presented by Swedish investigators at the congress. The Swedish researchers had cultured the polio virus in laboratory monkeys from secretions of three asymptomatic human cases, a method that experimentally confirmed earlier epidemiological suggestions

about the important role of hidden carriers in spreading polio.[113] In December 1912, when federal epidemiologist Wade H.
Frost analyzed this conference for the Public Health Service, he
was more impressed with Rosenau's studies. These were "careful
and masterly epidemiological investigations," he wrote. The
Swedish researchers, Frost noted, had shown that nonsympto-
matic polio cases were probably common, but Rosenau's work
demonstrated that the stable fly was "an important or even necessary factor in the transmission of poliomyelitis."[114] Experimental
work by Frost and John F. Anderson at the federal Hygienic
Laboratory reinforced Rosenau's theory, and other health officials, repeating these experiments in their own laboratories, announced their results triumphantly in the daily press.[115]

During the 1916 epidemic officials turned to entomologists
for expert advice. "PLEASE RECOMMEND AT ONCE ENTO-
MOLOGIST AND SALARY TO MAKE SURVEY OF FLIES IN
NEW YORK CITY" Haven Emerson telegramed Ephraim Felt,
New York's state entomologist.[116] In early August Emerson met
with the region's prominent insect experts, including the state
entomologists of New York, New Jersey, and Connecticut. This
conference strongly impressed Felt, who later explained to Hermann Biggs that their discussion had shown "rather clearly that
human carriers of infantile paralysis could hardly be held responsible for all cases and there was considerable evidence in
favor of some insect or insects being carriers."[117] Furthermore,
Felt argued that polio's epidemiological pattern reinforced the
fly theory of transmission, and he reiterated the striking evidence against direct contagion: there were no polio cases among
the thousands of children in the city's public institutions, nor had
any hospital attendant or physician developed the disease.[118]

Emerson hired Charles Brues from the Bussey Institute at
Harvard to study the New York City epidemic for two months.[119]
After an extensive survey of the role of insects and other possible
sources of infection, Brues attacked Flexner's contact theory.
"One fact that seems perfectly clear," he wrote, "is, that . . .
where large numbers of persons are crowded in congested dwellings, there is no tendency toward a rise in the incidence of poliomyelitis." This fact, he wrote, "offers poor support to the view

that these cases have been contracted as a result of contact with children suffering from the disease."[120] An insect theory, he argued, was a more appealing epidemiological explanation. Brues was less enthusiastic about the idea that the infection was spread by the housefly as a mechanical carrier, for the theory that the fly contaminated food with the polio virus as it did with the germ of typhoid fever was "an assumption not supported by any evidence." But he did emphasize the possible role played by biting insects like stable flies and fleas.[121] Although Brues did not reach a firm conclusion about any insect, the enthusiastic city health department published his long report as a separate pamphlet and distributed it to the public.[122]

The fly theory became the target of much scientific debate. Simon Flexner had long harbored doubts about a simple link between flies and polio. But as a prominent scientific researcher who had established the viral etiology of polio a few years earlier, Flexner was frequently called upon to offer his opinions on all aspects of the nature, control, and treatment of the epidemic. His replies were usually careful and conservative. In July 1916, during a widely reported meeting on the disease at the New York Academy of Medicine, Flexner stressed that the polio virus had never been found in human blood (unlike the agent of yellow fever, for example). How, then, he wondered, could the polio virus travel to the brain and spinal cord after the bite of an infected fly? In an article published in the *Journal of the American Medical Association* Flexner was even less enthusiastic about the fly transmission theory, but he did not explicitly attack official anti-fly campaigns.[123]

Undaunted, Emerson's health officers continued their efforts, and anti-fly work became a major part of the public health campaign against polio during the summer months of 1916. The link between filth and flies seemed clear, and cleanup campaigns were frequently justified as a way to rid a community of fly-breeding refuse. Pennsylvania's state health commissioner was one of the theory's most fervent proponents. In response to diverse outbreaks of polio in 1916, Dixon ordered a statewide cleanup, particularly in "built-up communities," and urged the Pennsylvania public to take proper care of handling garbage so as to prevent the breeding of flies and the "trailing of putrid substances by flies and other insects to the food of children." Similarly, a health officer in East Orange, New Jersey, used the threat of an epidemic to enforce more strictly antimanure regulations.[124]

Although most researchers linked the spread of polio to the biting stable fly, public health officials warned the public against all kinds of flies. A Newark official announced that "some insect" was bringing infected material to humans "which develops into polio," and although only horse and cattle flies and not the housefly bite, the public should "swat them all."[125]

The practical side of the anti-fly campaign, and its connection between dirt and disease, appealed not only to health officers but also to lay health reformers. In mid-August Edward Hatch, Jr., head of the Fly-Fighting Committee of the New York Merchants Association, which had led numerous anti-fly campaigns, blamed the epidemic on new subway construction. Builders had left large deposits of manure to keep pipes from freezing. The manure piles, which were not properly covered up, Hatch warned, were breeding flies in the millions, becoming a "large factor in infantile paralysis." Emerson, in response, said that the sanitary bureau and the city's new entomologist would investigate the claim.[126]

Flies, officials assured the public, could easily be removed. Middle-class New Yorkers went into the streets at the urging of the Health Department and private agencies, swatting flies with enthusiasm. Department stores also readily adopted anti-fly slogans. Gimbels Department Store in Philadelphia promised that fly swatters and screens would "protect the children," for "one fly may cause a death in a household."[127] There were numerous proposed methods of fly prevention: the screen, the trap, and the fly swatter. In July 1916, the Washington Market Merchants Association suggested installing electric fans to deal with the fly problem; and Herman Horning, Philadelphia's city entomologist, suggested setting up giant fly traps in all the city's market places, each big enough to catch a million or so flies a day.[128]

The fly was a potent cultural symbol. In words and pictures enthusiastic health reformers emphasized the disgusting nature

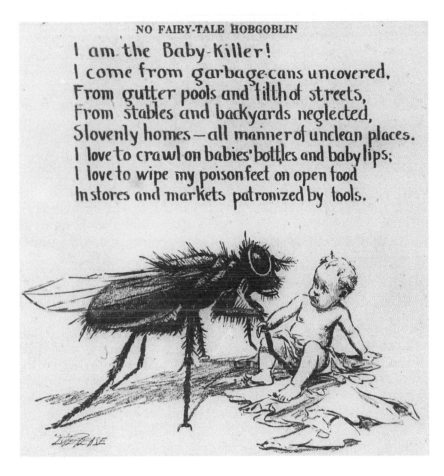

Fig. 8 Flies were blamed for the spread of children's diseases, June 1916
(*Newark Evening News*)

and appearance of this insect. In 1916 the woman's page of a
Newark paper illustrated this gruesome poem with a fly grin-
ning evilly at a child:

> I am the Baby Killer!
> I come from garbage-cans uncovered.
> From gutter pools and filth of streets,
> From stables and backyards neglected,

Slovenly homes—all manner of unclean places.
I love to crawl on babies' bottles and baby lips;
I love to wipe my poison feet on open food
In stores and markets patronized by fools.[129]

Flies were not inextricably linked to the slums; they could spread disease more or less randomly and unpredictably. The epidemiological clarification that the fly vector theory promised was particularly appealing in the case of polio. Some observers believed that the fly theory had solved the problem of explaining the appearance of polio cases in clean, suburban homes. Using the fly as a malleable sign of the violation of sanitary laws, officials tried to instruct both the middle-class and the poor in the laws of cleanliness. The fly, they stressed, crossed class lines while spreading dirt and disease. The editor of the *New York Times,* while acknowledging disagreements among scientists, urged New Yorkers not to "strengthen the ally of sickness," for the fly survived winters, rode in Pullman cars, and was no stranger to either Fifth Avenue or the tenements.[130]

More than simply providing a practical method, the anti-fly theory appeared to clarify the thorny issues of responsibility for the spread of disease. Flies could carry germs from the slums to the suburbs. "A wise mother screens the crib," warned Samuel Dixon, for "flies can carry the germs of typhoid fever and other diseases." There were, he announced, "thousands of children under one year who die annually" who could be saved if the fly could be eliminated.[131] Philadelphia official Wilmer Krusen pointed out that the disease appeared not only in the houses of the poor but also among the "moderately well-to-do." "We must all reiterate our warning[s] to watch out for flies, cook all foodstuffs, and clothe the child properly," he said.[132]

Even as this work offered officials practical and satisfying ways to deal with the disease, it also limited their role in the community. Despite the broad, sanitarian slant of anti-fly work, it in fact continued the narrowing of the sphere of public health work that proponents of the New Public Health had encouraged. Health reformers increasingly focused on homes rather than streets, and domestic hygiene rather than public sanitation. They tried to portray themselves as educators rather than regulators, although this definition did not hold up well under the stress of the 1916 epidemic.

Not all members of the public were convinced by this sanguine approach. Many continued to blame filth, pollution, and poverty as the source and cause of the epidemic. Anti-fly work became caught up in political struggles. The Staten Island Civic League sent letters to New York's governor, city mayor, and health commissioner; the league argued that scientists agreed the "germ of infantile paralysis" was spread by "flies feeding on filth," and thus the city should abandon its policy of handling city garbage so as to obtain a profit, and burn it instead.[133] One Philadelphia woman complained to her local paper: "instead of reclining back in office chairs, telling us mothers to be careful of flies, and keep our homes clean," the "health experts down in City Hall" should stop "talking about covered garbage pails and flies and find out how often their men collect the garbage that breeds the flies."[134] And a New York mother, after reminding her city's mayor of the panic among mothers vacationing with their children outside the city, urged him to investigate "pest holes" where flies came into direct contact with poor sufferers and their excrement.[135]

Some citizens were suspicious of the motives behind their health department's enthusiastic attack of the fly. In August, Wilmer Krusen, warning that "the fly, the open garbage can and the dirty street are the greatest enemies of the children at present," urged Philadelphia to pay for additional quarantine enforcers and sanitary inspectors.[136] By employing a number of potential city voters in active preventive work, fly campaigns were good publicity for health departments. Some Philadelphians, however, were less enthusiastic; one citizen complained that Krusen's hiring of extra "scoundrelly" inspectors was a tactic more relevant to political maneuvering for the next city election than the prevention of disease.[137]

Overall, however, the public seems to have accepted the anti-fly theory, and some even used flies as object lessons for children. In mid-July public complaints reached the local newspaper after a dead dog had been left on a city street in Newark for two days, gathering flies. Angry residents placed lighted candles on the curb and a sign in thick black letters: "Beware of the Dog." Parents took their children there and warned them that "if they went too near the dog they might contract infantile paralysis, like other little children, and die." According to one report, as the children stood around the dog they "saw the swarm of flies spiral upward and sail away in their thousand directions. And the children fled in terror."[138]

While anti-fly campaigns narrowed the focus on the home as the appropriate locus for public health work, this emphasis may have also provided a stronger role for some women, as the home, seen as a sanitary haven, was threatened by germs from the street. Middle-class women from philanthropic associations and the settlement house movement could now expand their role to include that of sanitary expert, instructing immigrant women on how to protect their own families. Briefly, anti-fly work became part of the "municipal housekeepers" movement that provided an active role for female social reformers. Mrs. George A. Duning, the head of Pennsylvania's Women Suffrage Association, offered to help fight the 1916 epidemic by pressuring municipalities to pass public health laws and enforce them. Mrs. Carrie Chapman Catt of the National American Woman Suffrage Association cooperated with New York's health department by distributing sanitary leaflets. Other female health advocates also participated. Mrs. F. G. Hodgon, head of the Jefferson Market Committee, informed the public of the giant fly trap that had been installed during the summer of 1915.[139]

Flies, thus, had both professional and popular appeal. Unlike the polio virus, they were visible, and not only to the eye of a specialist with a powerful microscope and laboratory equipment. And unlike cats, dogs, or public library books, flies were everywhere. Their movements were unpredictable; they might have feasted on a refuse dump, on a dead horse in a Brooklyn canal, or on dirty milk and rotting food. They were a clear sign of unsanitary living conditions. If houses were clean they did not have flies; thus, flies were signs of individual irresponsibility and ignorance.

The fly theory focused attention on living conditions but not on water or food polluted by industry. Disease could endanger the inmates of tenements as the result of flies and poor sanitation, not the result of bad housing, grasping landlords, or poverty. Such public health work urged the reform of individual personal habits and the immediate domestic environment, rather than broad social change. Increasingly narrow and domestic, this approach focused on the home, defining an environment controllable by individual effort. Landlords had to ensure that ashes and garbage were properly collected, but tenants equally were expected to cover garbage cans and obey other municipal sanitary regulations. By screening windows and forbidding the consumption of street candy parents could do something practical to protect their children, although the disease continued to appear in homes presumed "safe." And officials, as expert educators and guardians of public health, having cleaned the streets, could now focus on teaching individuals their civic responsibilities.

The 1916 polio campaign must be understood in the context of Progressive reform. In this era, middle-class men and women tried to use legislative power as well as moral persuasion to "clean up" urban social problems. The city, they believed, was both exhilarating and threatening, but its dirt—moral and physical— had to be removed before it could be a healthy place for either the poor or the middle-class to live. Reformers believed that regulation was not enough; the behavior of individuals had to be altered. Through education and science they hoped to transform family, home, community, and finally society.

To achieve this, health reformers—whose ranks included social workers, physicians, and suffragists—drew on the expertise of the social and medical sciences. In their conception of the proper direction of public health work, however, they shifted uneasily between an environmental explanation linking poverty with disease, and one based on the idea of individual

responsibility and the randomness of the germ theory. Polio
was explained in both terms of the traditional filth theory and
the concepts of modern bacteriology. Even the most up-to-date
scientists, who tended to support a theory of personal contact
in disease transmission, mixed their anlayses of the epidemic
with dust and fomites, older symbols of disease.

The public health campaigns against the 1916 polio epidemic
demonstrated a concern with place, not just as the source of
infection but also as the means of protection from disease. Disease and victim were identified by place; a sick child's home and
neighborhood were thus used to designate their probable safety
from infection. Officials, trying to link public and private
spheres, argued that members of the public should responsibly
keep their own households clean and follow sanitary guidelines;
this left officials with the task of public sanitation such as street
cleaning and garbage removal. The 1916 epidemic did focus
some attention on the terrible conditions of the urban immigrant
poor, but citizens tended to worry more about the immediate
sanitation of the domestic environment, particularly aesthetic
problems of dirt and smells. The idea that flies were spreading
the disease linked these traditional fears with the tools and concepts of modern science.

New Public Health theory and practice, thus, did not resolve
the role of the environment and the extent of individual responsibility. Nor did science offer objective ways to judge the extent of
danger of different kinds of behavior, people, and places. The
germ theory and bacteriological techniques allowed some health
officials to concentrate their efforts on the individual. But an
older emphasis on environmental sanitation persisted, and sanitation and education efforts were directed at immigrant families
presumed to require sanitary instruction. The public health campaigns against polio reflected traditional fears of dirt and
fomites, immigrants and the poor. "I am very seriously troubled," Emerson wrote to Flexner as the 1916 epidemic began to
decline, "as are many people in the city government, by the tendency shown in many places in and outside of the city to a distinction between what is safe for the children of the poor and what is
safe for the children of the well to do."[140]

Anti-polio campaigns made visible popular sentimental ideas: the health of country air and its inverse, the dangerous dirty city; the innocent child victim and its careless parents. The disease appeared especially frightening due to the unusual susceptibility of both rich and poor children; the few adults affected were not integrated into public health campaigns or discourse. Health officers also knew that they were generally unable to identify healthy infected carriers. But they continued to target groups of immigrants, the poor, and the dirty—groups they expected to be both victims and carriers. The contradictory evidence from epidemiological fieldwork and laboratory experiments reinforced rather than contradicted these efforts.

CHAPTER THREE

The Promise of Science: Polio and the Laboratory

Late in 1916 in a letter to a New York State official the secretary of a Manhattan physicians' group complained about the "domination of the laboratory man in the profession." The recent polio epidemic, he reflected, had shown the uselessness of "laboratory men" compared to the skills of "old fashioned medical men" such as himself.[1] "The spectacle of experimentalists posing as practitioners," another physician agreed, was "reflected in our present day medical graduates facile of experiment and blind at the bedside. The community is not served best so."[2]

During the 1916 epidemic daily newspapers reported regular meetings among scientists and clinicians to discuss the disease. Private physicians attacked these conferences, some for their lack of resolution, others for their exclusionary policies. *"These distinguished physicians represent the Trust element in the profession,"* a Brooklyn man complained in a letter to the mayor of New York City, a group, he believed, that was "responsible for turning out medical men on the public with only a theoretical knowledge of their business." "It is this element," he explained, "that excludes the family physician from hospitals."[3]

Patients and physicians in the early twentieth-century United States were hopeful that the new scientific medicine would enable physicians to diagnose, treat, and prevent disease with new precision. Science in the Progressive era was seen as an objective, potent, and transforming tool, best employed by experts. But in the case of polio the promise of new medical sciences remained frustratingly unfulfilled. The integration of scientific medicine's concepts and methods into medical practice became part of the debate over who was to be the new expert in managing polio.

What was to be the proper relationship of the laboratory to bedside practice? Should the laboratory be the healer's handmaiden or the decisive source of medical knowledge and authority? Patients wondered how such decisions would influence their treatment and their relationship with practitioners. Physicians feared that their clinical judgment would be replaced by complex technology in the hands of laboratory specialists. Nor were physicians at one on this question. For medical teaching and professional careers, in many cities the increasing importance of the modern hospital, offering ambitious clinicians access to the laboratory and diverse clinical material, had begun to reinforce differences between specialists and general practitioners.[4] Tensions between physicians and laboratory scientists were heightened during the 1910s and 1920s as the roles of private physician, hospital clinician, and pathologist were becoming increasingly separate. And the status of the general practitioner, unattached to hospital or clinic, grew increasingly precarious.[5]

Members of the public and the medical profession who turned to laboratory science debated its worth as resource and authority. In the following chapter I explore the ways patients explained epidemic polio by using the tools and ideology of science. Here I examine the debate among hospital clinicians, private physicians, and laboratory scientists over two aspects of medical practice: polio diagnosis and polio therapy.

The new sciences of bacteriology and immunology had provided medical practitioners with tools for the diagnosis, treatment, and prevention of numerous diseases. By the 1910s, European and American scientists had produced a range of immunological therapies, including antitoxins against diphtheria, tetanus, and rabies, and vaccines for cholera, typhoid, plague, and yellow fever. Where a disease's etiology was more complicated, there were also experimental "mixed" stock vaccines, as well as "autogeneous" sera that could be tailored to the individual bacterium of a sick patient.[6] Diagnostic techniques, based on tracing antibody reactions, included skin reaction tests for diphtheria and tuberculosis and blood tests for syphilis and typhoid.

These tools offered physicians the ability to identify the etiological agents of disease, pinpoint and treat infected individuals, and prevent disease among the uninfected. They also inspired in many a more general faith in the laboratory as the solution to health problems. First, find the germ; everything else would follow. But these tests were not straightforward; they demanded bacteriological and immunological knowledge and skill. And who was to interpret their results: the family doctor, the hospital clinician, or the specialist trained in pathology and bacteriology? The increasing reliance on these technologies threatened to redefine medical practice and diminish the private physician's stature. Although physicians accepted the premise of the new scientific medicine—that the laboratory should be an important standard in developing and testing clinical insights—they were nonetheless uncertain of the place to which this relegated clinical experience and judgment. "If the mystery of disease has largely been destroyed through the detection of its microscopical agents," reflected one physician who outlined "Fifty Years of Medical Progress" in 1916, "so has the halo of miraculous power that formerly encircled the brow of the erudite magister of the healing art."[7]

By 1909 the polio germ had been established, and doctors turned to the laboratory for tools to identify and treat the infected. Clinicians analyzed spinal fluid obtained by a spinal tap (or lumbar puncture as it was formally termed) and, amid a host of proposed polio treatments, tested an anti-polio serum made of the blood of patients who had recovered from the disease. But, I argue, the development and application of these tools were complicated and problematic. Physicians judged the aptness of diagnostic and therapeutic techniques by the context in which they were to be used. Friends and family of a patient thus could potentially play a significant role in determining diagnostic and therapeutic methods, particularly in the case of this frightening and confusing disease. And, unlike those who developed the techniques, not all patients or practitioners shared the same understanding of the nature of the disease or ways to judge their results.

Since the 1890s American physicians had at their disposal numerous clinical reports of polio cases. These studies, however, mostly discussed only a few patients, without reference to similar reports, and were scattered throughout the medical literature. In 1912, researchers at the Rockefeller Institute's Hospital, which had opened two years earlier, published a major review of the clinical aspects of the disease, based on almost two hundred patients, the first substantial clinical investigation of the disease in the United States. Although Francis Peabody, George Draper, and Alphonse Raymond Dochez were unable to explain many of polio's puzzling epidemiological features, these authors outlined the major practical and conceptual issues raised in trying to diagnose and treat the disease. They reminded physicians that polio's infectious agent was not bacterial but a filterable virus, which was highly resistant to freezing and carbolic acid but could be destroyed, in the laboratory at least, by heat and hydrogen peroxide. While therapy remained primarily symptomatic, scientists in France, Germany, and the United States had found a neutralizing substance in the blood of both humans and monkeys; this promised the possibility of developing a polio serum or antitoxin.[8]

Integrating clinical, pathological, and experimental findings, the Rockefeller investigators urged physicians to adopt an expansive definition of the disease. Despite its visible defining symptom, paralytic polio was not just a disease of the central nervous system but a "general infection." The virus must "rest for a time" in other organs, the authors of the report suggested, and then was probably conveyed to spine and brain by the blood stream, although the virus had not been consistently found in the blood of either humans or monkeys. The authors echoed their Rockefeller research colleagues' belief that nose and throat secretions remained vital to explaining its spread from person to person.[9] Early diagnosis was critical, for as

Swedish epidemiologist Ivar Wickman had shown, polio epidemics could be spread by patients with the disease but without paralysis or any symptoms at all. Wickman's work suggested that the clinician's eye could be insufficient to detect the fleeting signs of the disease's early stages, which were usually overlooked even by "intelligent parents." Clinical observation had to be careful and attentive; there was, for example, no distinctive rash, as some physicians had suggested. Beyond the clinician's eye, the analyses of body products such as blood and spinal fluid were quite useful, but the authors warned that the infecting organism was too small to be seen or cultured, a point soon contested by Rockefeller virologists.[10] Overall, their study suggested that clinical observation remained the most promising, for laboratory tests of body products were confusing and difficult to evaluate. The authors' detailed descriptions of the disease's clinical features reflected many physicians' beliefs that the only clear way to identify the disease was from the bedside, through the experienced eye of the clinician.

This emphasis on bedside observation and the clinician's eye differed substantially from the approach of contemporary laboratory scientists who studied the polio virus in experimental animals, mostly monkeys. Simon Flexner had gained international prominence with his experimental work on the polio virus. As early as America's first major polio epidemic in New York City in 1907, Rockefeller scientists had begun extensive virological studies of polio under his direction. Flexner, however, kept his experimental work strictly separate from his colleagues' clinical studies. During their work for the 1912 report, for example, although Hospital researchers Peabody, Draper, and Dochez wished to compare the appearance of the polio virus in humans to monkeys, they were denied access to Rockefeller laboratory resources.[11]

Through his polio experiments Flexner helped introduce polio's etiological agent, identify "neutralizing substances," and establish Rhesus monkeys as useful experimental animals for polio research. Flexner, arguing that the nose and mouth were the disease's portals of entry, paid little attention to contemporary findings of either the virus in the intestines or the gastrointestinal symptoms noted by many doctors. Downplaying evidence of the virus in the bloodstream, he also argued that the virus traveled directly from the nose and mouth to the central nervous system. His intransigence and influence among American virologists, later historians have argued, may have delayed understanding of polio's complex clinical and epidemiological features for at least a generation.[12] Flexner's emphasis on interpreting polio through animal experiments reflected his belief that laboratory research, not clinical or epidemiological observation, offered the most promising path in polio research.[13]

THE NEED FOR DIAGNOSIS

Both physicians and lay citizens found it difficult to link paralytic cases. In 1905 Ivar Wickman's suggestion that mild cases played a major role in spreading the disease had reinforced the importance of precise and accurate diagnosis of polio in the early stages.[14] But how were physicians to identify these cases, when the early symptoms of the disease—stiff neck, fever, nausea, and weakness—characterized other more common children's illnesses?[15]

During epidemics, as medical historians have shown, physicians dealing with a disease with powerful social and political consequences, have tended to employ flexible diagnostic categories. Under such circumstances doctors have hesitated to label a patient with a morally suspect disease such as syphilis or identify an individual or a household as the source of tuberculosis, cholera, or plague.[16] Similarly, American clinicians found in the ubiquitous early symptoms of polio considerable diagnostic latitude. Physicians, seeking to calm parents, could offer alternative diagnoses of suspicious symptoms, including acute gastroenteritis, ptomaine poisoning, pneumonia, meningitis, typhoid fever, and rheumatism, conditions that doctors may have felt more confident in treating.[17] Such flexibility, however, tended to blur medical confidence in polio as a distinct entity. In 1909 Minnesota public health officer Herbert Winslow Hill noted that some local physicians were using the term polio to categorize a variety of ills.

Hill offered as evidence one doctor who had identified fifty-six cases as polio. At least fifty-one of them were in fact tonsillitis, Hill believed, but the physician insisted that the cases "constituted a series of increasing severity, all being poliomyelitis but in different stages."[18]

As polio outbreaks became more common, practitioners sought fast and effective diagnostic techniques. After all, ignoring or misdiagnosing a case of polio could endanger a whole community and severely damage a physician's reputation. A U.S. Public Health Service officer argued that prompt diagnosis was critical for not only preventive measures but also effective therapy.[19] Waiting for the appearance of more definite signs such as paralysis could be too late; many physicians believed that to achieve the greatest efficacy of the limited therapy available it must be applied in the earliest stages of the disease.[20]

But diagnosing polio posed practical and theoretical difficulties. The polio virus, unlike the etiologic agents of diphtheria or typhoid, was too small to be seen under an ordinary microscope and too difficult, perhaps impossible, to cultivate. Although European and American scientists had established the viral etiology of polio by 1909, physicians continued to disagree about the nature and shape of the virus. Some years after the agent of polio had been shown to be a virus, New York City's health commissioner argued that "notwithstanding their many experiments, full proof is wanting that the minute organism described by Flexner and Noguchi . . . is the specific cause of polio."[21]

The search for polio diagnostic techniques centered around laboratory tools for identifying the microorganism. The laboratory, after all, had provided specific tests for diseases such as typhoid fever, diphtheria, and tuberculosis, including complement fixation, urine and blood analysis, growing microorganisms in various culture media, and assessing the reactions of experimental animals injected with infected material. Pathology was becoming a distinctive speciality; its techniques were available for hospital clinicians and private physicians who chose to send products to a private laboratory. Some public health departments also established their own laboratories. By 1916 New

York City's public health laboratory had developed a national reputation, although some city physicians remained resistant to municipal interference into their diagnosis and care of private patients.[22]

During polio epidemics physicians in the Northeast turned to the work of laboratory scientists at the Rockefeller Institute. But most of this work was of no immediate help to either the private practitioner or the health official. Flexner used expensive and complex technology, including monkeys that were costly and difficult to handle. His diagnostic techniques dealt almost exclusively with spinal cord products—injecting pieces of spinal cord from suspected polio cases into monkeys and waiting to see if paralysis developed—although Flexner acknowledged that it was difficult for private practitioners to obtain permission to perform autopsies on their polio patients. Flexner's view of the virus traveling directly to the nervous system meant that he rarely examined other pathological material that might have been easier for private physicians to obtain, such as blood or urine.[23]

But physicians were not limited to Rockefeller techniques. They could draw on their own clinical experiences and their senses. They could use a microscope and simple culture media; they could send body products to private and public laboratories for analysis; and they could select from the diagnostic techniques developed by laboratory scientists. Still, unlike most laboratory scientists, their choices were structured by the context of medical care. The diagnostic process involved both patient and physician and depended on their shared faith in laboratory science as resource and authority. A patient's class, the place of diagnosis (bedside, hospital ward, or laboratory), and lay and medical ideas of disease helped determine which diagnostic methods were employed, to whom they were given, and the way their results were interpreted.

In the 1910s the most promising tool for diagnosing polio was examination of a patient's spinal fluid. Doctors obtained spinal fluid by puncturing the skin between vertebrae, usually the third and fourth, with a needle and extracting between ten and thirty cubic centimeters of spinal fluid.[24] The fluid was then inspected

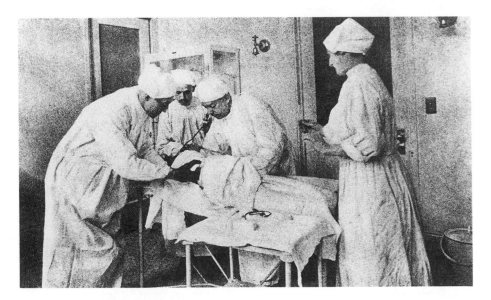

Fig. 9 A spinal tap performed in a New York City hospital during the 1916
epidemic (Haven Emerson, *A Monograph on The Epidemic of Poliomyelitis* [*Infantile Paralysis*] *in New York City in 1916. Based on the Official Reports of the Bureaus of the Department of Health* [New York: Department of Health, 1917])

by the naked eye and through a microscope; where possible, it
was spun through a centrifuge to obtain sediment.

The method to obtain the fluid, lumbar puncture, was itself
controversial. This difficult and potentially dangerous technique was used mainly for neurological conditions, for in most
nonneurological illnesses a spinal tap is "dry." The pressure of
the fluid was often difficult to control, and physicians had to be
careful not to puncture a vein. Nor was the technique completely safe. The amounts of fluid withdrawn were by today's
standards quite large: in one study a researcher withdrew between 20 and 100 cubic centimeters from twenty-seven children
under five.[25]

In an era when many physicians were unfamiliar with even
the hypodermic syringe, pathologists argued (with some reason) that both obtaining the fluid and testing it were techniques
often beyond the ability of the average physician. A report is-

sued by a New York committee on polio concluded that lumbar puncture was "a process requiring some technical skill, and should be attempted only by a specially trained physician."[26] "Lumbar puncture for diagnosis," U.S. Public Health Service officers John Anderson and Wade Frost agreed, "is hardly justifiable, however, unless some consideration of the safety, either of the patient or of the community, makes an accurate diagnosis of special importance."[27] The use of lumbar puncture had been widely discussed since a meningitis epidemic in New York City in 1907. But eight years later New York pathologists Phebe DuBois and Josephine Neal noted that few hospital staff members knew how to do the procedure properly.[28]

Still, unlike Flexner's analysis of spinal cord material, spinal fluid was at least an option for physicians dealing with live patients. Its analysis did not involve laboratory animals, and the concept of lumbar puncture was already familiar to physicians who had used the technique during the 1907 meningitis epidemic.[29] During the 1916 epidemic the New York City Health Department incorporated the technique into city hospital routine and used lumbar puncture as means of identifying obscure cases. Health officials put suspicious cases under quarantine restrictions until the results of analysis indicated whether the patient had the disease.[30] The diagnosis of polio "has received a tremendous boost during the last summer," one New York official commented in 1917. "The old idea prevalent among the general profession" that a polio case is defined only by signs of paralysis or muscle weakness "received a rather severe jolt," he argued, and the change was, he believed, "largely due to the widespread use of the lumbar puncture needle and the examination of spinal fluid."[31]

THE MURKY CLARITY OF SPINAL FLUID

Unlike diagnostic tests for diphtheria, tuberculosis, and typhoid fever, spinal fluid analysis for polio was complicated and unclear.[32] Even physicians with the skills to handle these tools frequently found their results confusing. Furthermore, analysis subsequent to the puncture was not uncomplicated. Spinal fluid analysis required not just a microscope but also a centrifuge to obtain sediment from the fluid. When the sediment from the fluid was cultured, there were no simple microorganisms to grow and no clear antibody reaction test. Continuing debates over fluid analysis suggest that the notion of polio as a viral disease was not fully accepted. There remained a number of contenders for polio's etiologic agent, including a bacterial diplococcus and the filterable virus, which Flexner and his colleague Noguchi claimed to have cultured in 1913. Nor were researchers confident that Flexner and Noguchi's "globoid body" was the microorganism of polio.[33]

Even after European and American scientists had established that polio's etiologic agent was not a bacterium physicians continued to experiment with the techniques developed for testing bacterial organisms. In 1910 a Kansas City physician, for example, tried to culture spinal fluid that had been injected into guinea pigs, rabbits, chickens, and two Rhesus monkeys.[34] Some years later, despite the controversial and inconclusive results of such tests, the *Journal of the American Medical Association* published a series of articles whose authors heatedly debated the "bacteriology of polio."[35]

Spinal fluid could be assessed by the naked eye. One physician noted an increase of white blood cells, which could be seen by either the naked eye or a pocket magnifying lens, and when he put a test tube in a dark room with artificial light he saw "dustlike little specks."[36] In fact, the existence of spinal fluid itself in a patient suggested a neurological condition. Spinal fluid from polio patients was also distinctive: unlike fluid in most cerebrospinal disorders, it was clear rather than cloudy. However, fluid from patients with tubercular meningitis was also clear, and only identifying the tubercle bacillus made the diagnosis certain. During epidemics of meningitis this confusion was increased.[37]

Unable to identify a distinct organism, physicians resorted to testing polio patients' spinal fluid for a variety of organic substances.[38] Researchers inferred meaning from chemical reactions and linked them to changes in their patients' bodies.

Pathologists DuBois and Neal, for example, assumed that an increase in the globulin content of spinal fluid demonstrated inflammation of the meninges, "and we have never had reason to doubt it."[39] These tests were based on those used for other pathological materials: Noguchi's work with syphilis had suggested the importance of assessing globulin content. Other tests included the albumin content (a test more typically applied to urine), reactions to a given chemical compound (Fehling's solution was popular), and the size, number, and type of cells found in the fluid.[40]

But researchers often did not agree about the significance of various chemical reactions. In November 1915 the *American Journal of Diseases of Children* published a major article on spinal fluid analysis, which, despite its detail, reached no clear conclusions. The author, Harry L. Abramson, was the head of New York City's Bureau of Laboratories. Abramson, who had worked with polio patients for four years, had forty-seven samples from twenty-six patients. He outlined the routine of fluid analysis: calculating the amount and gross appearance of the fluid; straining the fluid's sediment after centrifuging it; making an estimated cell count; sketching the types of cells and noting any unusual ones. He cultured this sediment, searched for organisms, and inoculated it into guinea pigs. The fluid's chemical content was assessed for albumin and globulin and its ability to reduce Fehling's solution.[41] Abramson also emphasized the importance of a clinical history, but he concluded that "examination of the spinal fluid is the most important factor in clearing up the diagnosis in abortive and preparalytic cases."[42]

Even with the skills to attempt such analysis, researchers found its results confusing. This ambiguity left space for clinical skills and insight in defining polio and became part of the debate over the proper role of the laboratory in medical practice. Critics compared the laboratory's ambiguous results to the clarity of polio's clinical signs. In 1910 Edward Mayer, a Pittsburgh physician, criticized the usefulness of lumbar puncture by comparing polio's "definite" clinical signs to the confusing results of fluid analysis: "Is this slight lymphocytosis with subsequent clearing of fluid and constant increase of polymorphonuclear leukocytes characteristic of poliomyelitis only? In other words, I cannot see in what way it makes the diagnosis any more definite than the excessive perspiration, the irregular tremor, the irritability and extreme prostration, the frequent suppression of urine, etc., which mark the disease before paralysis."[43]

Even laboratory workers stressed the importance of a good clinical history. DuBois and Neal, for example, found a clinical history indispensable to differentiate tubercular meningitis from polio "because the chemical and microscopic pictures are so frequently identical in the two conditions." Polio, they noted, could usually be distinguished by the sudden onset of preparalytic symptoms, including a high temperature that suddenly dropped, a stiff neck, and other slight signs that often took "careful questioning to elicit."[44] Spinal fluid examination, Harry Abramson agreed, was "of the greatest help" in diagnosing atypical and nonparalytic cases. But, he warned members of the New York State Medical Society, "you should not make a diagnosis of poliomyelitis on the examination of the spinal fluid alone," for similar fluid results could be obtained from cases of typhus fever and meningitis. "Therefore," he concluded, "one must add the laboratory findings to the clinical picture in arriving at a proper diagnosis."[45]

THE CONTEXT OF DIAGNOSIS

Lumbar puncture could be employed at any stage of polio, but practitioners admitted that as their patients began to improve it was difficult to justify the procedure. In 1910 a Canadian physician told Flexner about an unusual case of two infected children from the same family. But, he added, "I regret that I cannot get any fresh spinal fluid as the relatives object to further puncture." Flexner, in reply, agreed that he could well understand the doctor's hesitation in attempting puncture, but he hoped that it would be "just possible . . . as to propose it." Flexner implicitly admitted the fears of many patients as he reminded the physician that "in children, of course, the carrying out of the puncture is almost painless, and especially after a whiff or two of chloroform or ethyl chloride." But the mother of the children in question nonetheless refused.[46]

During this period many physicians, distrusting such intrusive procedures, were not surprised that their patients were also suspicious. In 1910, after reading an article by Flexner in the *Journal of the American Medical Association,* Edward Mayer reminded the *Journal's* editor and other physicians that if lumbar puncture were performed before paralysis occurred it "may be blamed by the relatives for the succeeding paralysis." The changes in the fluid were, in any case, Mayer believed, not as definitive as changes in blood counts that revealed an "abnormal number of lymphocytes."[47]

In his reply, Flexner defended this technique. He agreed that doctors should "exercise a great caution so that a misunderstanding does not arise on the part of the friends of the patient" and advised that puncture "be not carried out in instances in which there is danger of such misinterpretation."[48] He emphasized the technique's clinical utility primarily in terms of its research potential. Lumbar puncture, he argued, provided the "one clinical method at present known for clearing up the diagnosis" of doubtful and atypical cases and distinguishing the symptoms of polio from the more familiar meningitis. The method also helped researchers learn more about abortive cases, particularly their frequency and "leading symptoms." But he cautioned that the technique should rarely be used by the "unskilled and inexperienced" because "in order to arrive at a diagnosis by this means laboratory knowledge is required, since the fluid . . . must be submitted to microscopic and chemical examinations." This, he believed, tended to "confine the method to the skillful" laboratory man.[49]

Flexner was confident that this technique's close association with the laboratory ensured use by only the trained and skillful. For him, accurate diagnosis was an end in itself or at least a critical research tool for defining clinical action. Physicians with limited access to elite urban hospitals and research facilities, however, were less often able to distance themselves from the desires and complaints of their patients' families. One doctor told Flexner that spinal fluid analysis was useless in his practice.

"The lumbar puncture would be fine if we had a laboratory," he explained, "but with no facilities and perhaps no one about who could tell the difference [between fluid changes] . . . it makes it look like cruelty to the kid."[50]

Some researchers based at city hospitals found patients, particularly working-class immigrants, difficult to convince. In 1915 DuBois and Neal summarized four years of meningitis research at the New York City Health Department Division of Laboratories; they warned that it took "tact and infinite patience to persuade some of the poor, ignorant, foreign patients to allow us to do [a lumbar puncture] . . . but usually if properly approached, they finally give in."[51] Sometimes the reluctance of such patients was seen as the result of their class and ethnicity; scientists suggested that these patients could not properly appreciate the power and capacity of laboratory science in modern American medicine. In 1910, Paul Lewis, director of the Henry Phipps Laboratory in Philadelphia, wrote to Flexner about a polio epidemic in the steel town of Bethlehem. The disease, Lewis explained, "so far has affected the poorer parts of the city; the patients are not of high intelligence and what we want most to do may be somewhat difficult, the matter of spinal puncture, that is."[52] Clearly, a doctor's ability to use lumbar puncture depended on the context. Health officials, specialists, and physicians with hospital appointments were more likely to use this technique than private practitioners.[53] Doctors dealing with polio victims in their own homes needed not only to obtain the parents' consent but also to convince them of this procedure's necessity. Not surprisingly, many clinicians expressed misgivings about this laboratory-oriented technique.

Nonetheless, some clinical specialists as well as pathologists urged general practitioners to use lumbar puncture despite its difficulties. In 1911 the eminent New York pediatrician Luther Emmett Holt, writing in the first issue of a new pediatric journal, argued that the introduction of the lumbar puncture in pediatric medicine was "as important an advance . . . as was the adoption of throat cultures in diphtheria." Clearly he hoped that spinal fluid analysis in cases of polio and meningitis would prove as promising in allowing for effective therapy as the throat culture had proven in relation to diphtheria antitoxin. Holt had performed lumbar puncture over a thousand times, but he agreed that it required "considerable skill" and "as strict asepsis as any surgical operation."[54]

But many doctors, remaining hesitant, continued to employ the full range of clinical diagnostic measures to diagnose the disease. In 1910, a physician outlined the symptoms of a Princeton freshman: malaise, headache, chills, constipation, pain at the back of the neck, and fatigue. The physician took his temperature, pulse, and respiration and examined his throat, abdomen, and reflexes. Unable to suggest a firm diagnosis, the doctor sent his patient to New York for the analysis of his urine, spinal fluid, and blood. By the third day "the diagnosis at this point was still obscure." The patient, he explained, "might have typhoid fever, gastro-intestinal toxemia, one of the more slowly developing meningitis, or poliomyelitis." A Widal blood test for typhoid proved negative, and finally a lumbar puncture was performed by extracting ten cubic centimeters of fluid. Flexner, who had been asked to examine the fluid, found that it resembled fluid taken from monkeys inoculated with the polio virus before the appearance of paralysis. The next day the patient developed a full-blown case of the disease, and his doctors extracted another ten cubic centimeters of fluid.[55]

For Holt the use of this technique had almost started to define the disease itself. He found it especially helpful in distinguishing atypical cases of polio from meningitis. But, he warned, as physicians grew "accustomed to place so much reliance on lumbar puncture" its products were becoming highly valued, and "the possibility of the existence" of polio or acute meningitis "with a normal fluid [was] . . . rather difficult to grasp." In one case Holt spent "several hours" looking for tubercle bacilli in the spinal fluid to prove that his patient, who had typical clinical symptoms of tubercular meningitis, had the disease. He was unable to find the relevant diagnostic indications. The child recovered and returned home and then died suddenly a month later.[56] Here, a commitment to laboratory analysis had discouraged a doctor from trusting his own clinical skills.

The laboratory did offer techniques for diagnosing polio.

These tools needed special skills, in both dealing with laboratory equipment and routine and in handling patients. But, more critically, they demanded a special faith in the usefulness of knowledge gained through laboratory analysis of body products. In the case of polio the laboratory did not "solve" the problem of diagnosis. Indeed, new laboratory methods provided too much information; researchers found many possible microorganisms and were uncertain how to assess their importance. And simultaneously the laboratory offered too little—broad, nonspecific chemical changes. Clinical observation remained vital to the diagnosis of this disease, but it did no more than underline medicine's inability to test or understand the complex etiology of polio. The debate over spinal fluid analysis suggests that the technique offered doctors flexibility at the same time that it directed them to rely more closely on laboratory techniques and integrate them as part of clinical practice.

POLIO THERAPIES

Just as the laboratory did not resolve the problems of polio diagnosis, so polio therapy similarly remained confusing. Debates over polio therapy reflected in part the shifting medical definition of the disease. In his *History of Poliomyelitis* historian John R. Paul has suggested that, as polio became more frequent in the last decades of the nineteenth century, American physicians reinterpreted the nature of the disease. Their definition shifted from a symptomatic model, based on clinical observations, to an anatomical pathological approach, stressing microscopic lesions found in the spinal cord, the intestines, and lymph nodes; to an experimental model, based on studies of the polio virus in humans and monkeys, showing the virus to be present in not only the spinal cord but also salivary glands and nasal secretions.[57] My analysis of medical reports in the 1910s suggests that all three models remained present in medical practice and that physicians were most skeptical of the usefulness of the experimental model.

In the 1910s Flexner and his Rockefeller colleagues tried to undermine earlier models of the disease based primarily on clinical and pathological observations. Yet their emphasis on understanding the disease through its reproduction in monkeys was not completely convincing to physicians dealing with sick human patients. Some doctors remained suspicious of analogies drawn between animals and humans; others were also not sure that finding the virus in various tissues explained the disease. Was polio, they asked, a general inflammation? a neurotropic infection? a distinct disease? or just a more severe form of other neurological disorders? These issues were based on the weight given to different sources of authority: the bedside, the autopsy room, and the experimental laboratory.

Conflicts over polio therapies in the 1910s reflected this confusion. And despite physicians' emphasis on the importance of early and accurate diagnosis to treat the patient and prevent epidemics, most available therapies were of limited efficacy. The various therapies employed and the fervent debates about their relative merits suggested diverse understandings of the workings of the disease itself; the discrepancies also made clear that some physicians had not abandoned the methods or theories of nineteenth-century medicine.

Physicians expected their treatments to make a difference. They looked to the laboratory for the development of immunological therapies that could be used swiftly and effectively at the bedside. Their expectations had been strengthened by the successful use of diphtheria antitoxin that had transformed the treatment of the otherwise often fatal children's disease. But they also relied on their clinical experience and knowledge. Instead of necessarily treating the disease "polio," when doctors identified fever, pain, and muscle weakness in their patients, they employed available therapies to treat those symptoms.

The techniques used in the 1910s by American physicians for treating polio patients ranged broadly, including counterirritation, bloodletting, cleansing the body, germ killing, and encouraging the production of antibodies. These treatments suggested that many physicians and patients had a rather confused understanding of the principles of immunology and the implications of the germ theory and showed moreover the continuing tradition of therapeutic practices and concepts from earlier eras. Healers, unwilling to jettison traditional therapies that both practitioner and patient had found helpful, looked both into the future and back to the past.

The debate over polio therapy grew particularly heated during this period because eminent scientific figures were reluctant to offer specific therapeutic suggestions. Flexner, for example, provided few clear leads from the results of his laboratory work. In 1910 George H. Simmons, the editor of the *Journal of the American Medical Association*, urged Flexner to overcome his reluctance to speculate about therapy and discuss "the principles underlying the treatment . . . because the question is a very live one at the present moment. . . . The great majority of the doctors who see these cases are at a loss to know what to do, and we should give them some suggestions if possible."[58] In response to the laboratory's limited answers, many physicians urged their colleagues to try any kind of therapy. During the 1916 epidemic a New York doctor argued that anything based on a sound rationale that was properly used should do no harm and "should theoretically do good . . . at least till we get something better."[59]

As recent studies of nineteenth-century American medical practice have shown, many physicians were loath to abandon the therapies of earlier generations, even as they espoused the ideals and methods of the new laboratory sciences.[60] Those who tried to treat polio patients during the early years of this century were similarly loyal to the therapies they had heard about in medical school, read in textbooks, and used successfully themselves. Although some of these practices were probably not typical of most private physicians, a few practitioners used treatments based on the theory of counterirritation: producing blisters by cupping the spine or using a mustard plaster.[61] In 1913 Philip F. Barbour, a Kentucky doctor, urged his colleagues to lessen the congestion of the cord by "any means available" and apply counterirritants "to bring the blood to the surface and away from the congested area."[62] In 1916 the South Carolina State Board of Medical Examiners included mild counterirritation through the use of mustard plasters in its acceptable answers to a question about polio therapy.[63]

Another continuity with therapies from an earlier era was
illustrated by physicians' concern with cleansing the body of
possible poisons through cathartic measures, usually based on
the model of polio as a disease affecting all parts of the body. As
polio was the result of excessive inflammation, one physician
argued, the rational treatment was depletion to eliminate the
unknown toxin, using bloodletting by leeches and catharsis.[64]
Although bloodletting was rarely discussed explicitly, other
methods reinforced the notion of the importance of cleansing
the body's toxic system. "The physician should realize that he is
dealing with a general infection involving all organs," wrote
another doctor, "and apply the same general principle of treatment as in other infectious diseases; hence the important principle of treatment is elimination."[65] These practitioners urged
their colleagues to use familiar purgatives such as calomel and
castor oil, as well as enemas and also hot packs for sweating out
toxins.[66]

Therapies were usually justified as symptomatic remedies.[67]
Physicians sought to temper their patients' fever, pain, vomiting, and diarrhea.[68] To produce distinct physiological changes
they used active chemical remedies, including bromides, chloral
hydrate, opiates, and coal tar preparations.[69] In 1917 New York
physician Walter Carr urged the use of mercuric chloride,
calomel, camphor, caffeine, sodium bromide, codeine, strychnine, and oxygen as indicated.[70] Doctors also warned that it was
important to build up the body as well. "Strychnine and all
other forms of tonics and general tonic medication should be
continued," Barbour argued.[71]

The use of these therapies clearly reflected pressure by anxious parents and the doctor's need to do something and be seen
doing something, particularly given a disease with such devastating possible consequences. For, as one physician warned, "mothers are overanxious when their children have this condition,
and they are willing to grasp at every straw, some of them
believing that the children will go through their whole lives with
a deformity." In fact, doctors needed to offer some kind of
therapy quickly, for parents, he argued, readily took "remedies
from each family that prescribes a remedy."[72] "The treatment

of the acute stage has received scant consideration," agreed an Omaha doctor. "If we can do nothing to modify the disease, certainly we can do something for the patient, and until the specific treatment is discovered it is the duty of the physician to institute proper treatment to meet the indications in the average case."[73]

Such practices were not without their critics. In his 1892 *Practices of Medicine* American clinician William Osler had argued that in treating polio the use of "blisters and other forms of counterirritation to the back is irrational and only cruel to the child."[74] In 1908 Massachusetts health officials doubted whether "much is accomplished by the administration of ergot and similar drugs or by blisters or other counter irritants applied to the back."[75] In 1910 a New York neurologist agreed that counterirritation was inadvisable "because it will interfere with the quiet rest of the patient on the back; because of the danger of the formation of bedsores; and, lastly, because it is more than doubtful whether it can do any good."[76] But these constant complaints suggest that these practices were continuing, whether sanctioned by science and elite professional approbation or not.

Physicians drew their therapeutic reasoning from clinical investigations as well as individual bedsides. A number of physicians adopted the notion of germ killing as a therapeutic principle. Disinfectants were widely believed to have therapeutic potential, not merely to keep germ-free children and houses but to cleanse the inside of the body as well.[77] "We might legitimately entertain the hope from our knowledge of the diffusion of formaldehyde within the system that soon we may be in possession of a substance which will be adequate to check the progress of the disease," wrote one physician.[78]

In 1908 Johns Hopkins Hospital researcher John Crowe, following a suggestion by Harvey Cushing, demonstrated that the disinfectant hexamethylenamin (popularly known as urotropin) appeared in the spinal fluid thirty minutes after intravenous injection. Practitioners hoped that this might offer therapeutic promise for neurological conditions. Crowe's study was widely quoted, and its implications expanded for both therapy and diagnosis.[79] A New York doctor administered urotropin "in the hope that formaldehyd[e] might be set free in the spinal cord."[80] In a letter to the editor published in the *Journal of the American Medical Association* in 1910, a Chicago physician urged that "in view of our desperate helplessness, a drug, backed as hexamethylenamin is by some experimental work, may be tried." He referred to the "well-established fact" that hexamethylenamin was excreted in the cerebrospinal fluid to explain the large doses he had given two patients at the onset of paralysis, and "in neither instance did the paralysis extend and both patients made good recoveries."[81] Health officials as well as private practitioners embraced this idea. Health officer Hill, though he admitted that Minnesota officials had "come to the end of our resources" and had "no inkling of how to prevent the disease," nonetheless advised the use of urotropin for children exposed to the disease or showing early symptoms.[82]

The idea of using a disinfectant to treat the disease, and to prevent its spread, was drawn from experimental work as well as clinical investigation. Physicians justified germ-killing therapies by turning to the results of Rockefeller scientists' laboratory work in which scientists used disinfectants to kill or render harmless the polio virus. After Flexner and Lewis noted the effectiveness of hydrogen peroxide, which destroyed the virus in vitro, a number of physicians used that disinfectant both as therapy and preventative.[83] Lewis Frissell, a New York physician, used a nasal spray of weak hydrogen peroxide solution "on the theory that the unknown organism might be eliminated though the nose."[84] A New York physician also urged the use of ammonium salicylate, due to its "known germicidal value."[85] On the fringes of such practices were suggestions such as that by William Benham Snow, editor of the *American Journal of Electrotherapeutics and Radiology*. During the 1916 epidemic, Snow reminded his colleagues that Flexner had shown that the polio microbe "only developed in the dark and that it was destroyed by light." He found, however, that neither the Rockefeller Institute nor the New York City's Health Department were interested in his theory of ultraviolet light as a germ-killing therapy. Told "there was nothing in it," he complained "that is the disposition of mind of those who are antagonistic and not willing to investigate but rather remain ignorant. . . . They seek blindly for some serum which may accomplish the impossible."[86]

Withdrawing spinal fluid also gained popularity as a therapeutic measure, based on both the idea of ridding the body of infected fluid and other poisons and also the clinical observation that removal of excessive fluid calmed the patient.[87] Pathologists DuBois and Neal claimed that even for meningitis cases that displayed unequivocal signs of the disease they performed lumbar puncture "as the withdrawal of the fluid seems to hasten recovery." Abramson recommended that physicians "withdraw as much [fluid] as will readily come, [but] minimizing the suddenness of withdrawal as much as possible." A clinician based at a New York City hospital believed that the technique was critical for polio patients, particularly during the acute state; if performed two or three times, he claimed it was the most appropriate therapy.[88]

Despite Flexner's reluctance, a few of his colleagues at the Rockefeller Institute did experiment with specific therapies during the 1916 epidemic. Simon J. Meltzer injected adrenalin after the withdrawal of spinal fluid and claimed that it aided the patient's recovery. He urged intraspinal injections of two cubic centimeters every six hours for at least four days. "We have definite evidence that the injections do no harm, and probable evidence that it does real good," he argued.[89] The editor of *New York Medical Journal* called for a fair trial of this therapy; he argued that adrenalin was "a direct activator of the antitoxic function" of the central nervous system, although he criticized its defenders' vague explanations of why it worked.[90]

By the second week of August 1916, Louis Ager, a Brooklyn pediatrician, was using adrenalin at Kingston Avenue Hospital under the direction of Meltzer.[91] This work, however, remained on the margins of elite professional interest. When Meltzer was not invited to a major conference of polio experts held at the College of Physicians and Surgeons, the editor of the *New York Times* complained that the "visitors were not enough interested in the administration of adrenalin to go to the hospital where good effects from its use are claimed, but they did refrain—and that is something—from scolding the doctor who suggested . . .

the novel remedy." The conference report, he continued, was disappointingly vague, and although the experts argued that "they are doing all that anybody could do, and that we should go on hoping for the best . . . the truth is that these gentlemen with the many degrees and titles know no more about infantile paralysis than does the medical profession in general."[92]

Physicians extended their faith in germicides to the working of antibodies. Human serum from those who had proven "immune" to the disease, some believed, might be able to kill polio germs. In 1910 health officials John F. Anderson and Wade H. Frost at the Hygienic Laboratory in Washington mixed virulent polio virus from Flexner's laboratory with this "normal" serum and found that three monkeys injected with the mixture did not develop paralysis. They suggested that "normal human serum may have a germicidal action on the virus of poliomyelitis." But they also believed that serum from patients who had recovered from the disease provided much greater "germicidal action."[93] During the 1916 epidemic, health officials' faith in serotherapy even expanded.

Physicians also suggested using therapy for one illness to treat another. During the 1907 New York epidemic of meningitis, a disease symptomatically similar to some forms of polio, Simon Flexner had successfully developed a diagnostic test based on spinal fluid analysis and an anti-meningitis serum. Many practitioners hoped that Flexner would develop a similar diagnostic technique and perhaps an anti-polio serum. Nor was serotherapy necessarily seen as etiologically specific. Some doctors also believed that Flexner's anti-meningitis serum might aid polio victims. As reports of polio cases began to increase after 1907, Flexner found that physicians often wrote to him asking for a supply of the anti-meningitis serum to be used on polio patients who had meningeal irritation as an "early and prominent feature."[94]

Physicians' search for polio treatments suggested an eclectic understanding of both the principles and practices of medicine by which they had been trained and which had altered substantially during their years as adult practitioners. Many physicians expressed a broad faith in the resources and potential of laboratory science, but this faith did not undermine other more conventional therapeutic practices and theories. While physicians sought modern laboratory tools, they continued to interpret their clinical experience in more traditional terms.

THE ANTI-POLIO SERUM

By the 1910s serum and vaccine production had become an integral part of health department work. New York City was known for its municipally funded laboratory that both tested and produced numerous immunologically based biological products for treating and preventing disease, including diphtheria and tetanus antitoxins, typhoid vaccines, and sera for pneumonia and meningitis.[95]

It was not surprising that citizens and physicians turned to serotherapy as a polio treatment. Diphtheria antitoxin developed by Emil Behring in 1891 had become a staple therapy promoted by major health departments such as New York City. It was one of the few clearly successful products of laboratory research efforts with potent power not only to prevent the disease but also to save dying children.[96] Many hoped that the laboratory would produce similar techniques for those children paralyzed and dying of this new disease.

These hopes were intensified by the knowledge that the efforts of health department officials, pursuing sanitary measures and health education, had not succeeded in halting polio epidemics. By 1910 American health officials had a new weapon against the disease: an anti-polio serum. In August 1916, the New York City Health Department began to publicize its use, and it was soon adopted by other cities' departments. Philadelphia's Wilmer Krusen promoted serum therapy as a critical preventive weapon and promised that polio would no longer be attacked "along strictly hygienic and sanitary lines." Now, he announced, "we strike at it with a force as great at its own."[97] Officials at the New York City Health Department assured the public that all potentially helpful therapies were being tested at city hospitals. Commissioner Haven Emerson noted that the

Table 1. Treatments Used at New York City Hospitals During 1916 Epidemic

Treatments	Willard Parker Hospital	Kingston Avenue Hospital	Riverside Hospital	Queensboro Hospital	Total
Serum	34	—	3	2	39
Adrenalin	2	11	23	—	36
Quinine	8	—	—	—	8
Horse serum	3	98	—	—	101
Diphtheria antitoxin	1	5	—	—	6
Lumbar puncture	405	328	158	65	956
Lumbar puncture and adrenalin	—	—	79	21	100
Serum X (special Jobling serum)	5	—	—	—	5
Auto-inoculation	5	29	—	—	34
Immune and normal serum	2	—	—	—	2
Spinal fluid	—	—	11	—	11
Immune serum	114	—	—	—	114
Normal blood citrated	2	—	—	—	2
Anti-meningitis serum	3	—	—	—	3
Anti-influenza serum	1	—	—	—	1
Symptomatic	1,489	563	929	102	3,083
Convalescent serum—spinal	—	9	—	—	9
Convalescent serum—muscular	—	6	—	—	6
Total	2,074	1,049	1,203	190	4,516

Source: Haven Emerson, *A Monograph on The Epidemic of Poliomyelitis (Infantile Paralysis) in New York City in 1916. Based on the Official Reports of the Bureaus of the Department of Health* (New York: Department of Health, 1917), 246.

four hospitals were treating polio by the "internal administration of urotropin, introspinal injections of adrenalin as recommended by Dr. S. J. Meltzer of the Rockefeller Institute, the injecting of immunizing serum from patients having had the disease, and the injection of normal serum of healthy persons."[98]

Developing a polio serum was difficult. The direct model was drawn from Flexner's work on meningitis therapy. His extremely successful anti-meningitis serum had been adopted by the city's Health Department as part of a new meningitis division. But laboratory workers were familiar with ways to cultivate the etiological agent of meningitis; polio's etiology was still a matter of scientific debate. True, Louis Pasteur had developed a vaccine for rabies in 1885 without having determined the agent of that disease, but the task for ordinary laboratory researchers was daunting.

Two kinds of anti-polio sera were used during the 1916 epidemic. The first, called normal serum, was discovered in 1910 by researchers at the Pasteur Institute in France; they suggested that in a general population there might be natural and inborn immunity to certain diseases and that normal serum made from the blood of adults could aid in treating and preventing disease. Or perhaps, as the epidemiological picture of epidemic polio seemed to confirm, adults naturally developed antibodies against the disease itself.[99] The use of normal serum raised questions of adults' immunity and resistance to polio. In 1913 the editor of the *Journal of the American Medical Association* suggested that normal serum "destroys or neutralizes the poliomyelitis virus." Its antibodies "on which resistance would seem to depend" were either "the expression of a natural, inborn immunity" or the result of a "latent infection" that does not develop to such an extent that "recognizable symptoms are produced."[100]

It was possible that the normal serum would also aid diagnosis of polio. Some practitioners wondered whether passive carriers—the healthy but infected—might be spreading polio. But there was no certain diagnostic test to identify such carriers and halt the spread of the disease. Pathologists DuBois and Neal suggested that the question of "natural immunity" had been "clearly demonstrated by means of the Schick test," which showed that diphtheria was spread by healthy infected children. They added that "analogy gives rational grounds for the belief that it also occurs in polio."[101]

A second kind of serum was developed from the blood of patients who had had polio and recovered. In 1910 both European and U.S. scientists, including Constanin Levaditi and Karl Landsteiner and Simon Flexner and Paul Lewis, had shown that when the serum of monkeys who had recovered from the disease was mixed with the polio virus and injected into a fresh monkey the serum failed to produce signs of the disease, suggesting that it had rendered the virus inactive. Soon scientists had demonstrated the same property with recovered human serum.[102]

The production of sera required laboratory facilities. Lacking such facilities, one doctor in 1916 injected patients with blood from healthy adults because most healthy adults appeared to be immune to polio and, he believed, the blood could offer food for the body's tissues and give the sick organism energy. "We get in whole blood the action of the injected phagocytic cells," he argued. In three cases the injection of this blood proved very successful, and he regarded "whole human adult blood" as superior to sera, both as a possible cure and preventative.[103]

Despite some interest in normal serum, recovered serum remained the most popular, made from the blood of either a person or monkey who had recovered from an attack of the disease. One problem with the clinical use of this serum was accumulating enough blood: recovered human victims before 1916 were relatively few and difficult to locate, and monkeys had little spare blood. Horses, the traditional animal for obtaining neutralized sera for other diseases, did not, unfortunately, seem to be affected by the disease.[104]

Abraham Zingher of the New York City Health Department became prominently associated with developing this form of polio therapy during the 1916 epidemic. In 1914 he had experimented with a measles serum, and later, while working at Manhattan's infectious diseases hospital, he began to experiment with recovered serum for polio.[105] Soon both city hospitals and some private practitioners were using serum. By mid-August, Philadelphia's city pathologist announced that he would try similar serum experiments. Numerous city departments called for volunteers to give blood.[106]

Reactions to the use of sera were mixed. New York City's Haven Emerson argued that the serum had not received a sufficient test and could not be pronounced generally effective for a long period of time. He compared cases of two children with identical conditions: the one who had received the serum had recovered; the other had also improved without the use of serum.[107] But other more enthusiastic supporters drew attention to the serum's link to the prestige of the new immunological sciences and eminent scientists and institutions. One physician noted that researchers had found that serum from a recovered patient or animal neutralized the virus in vitro and when

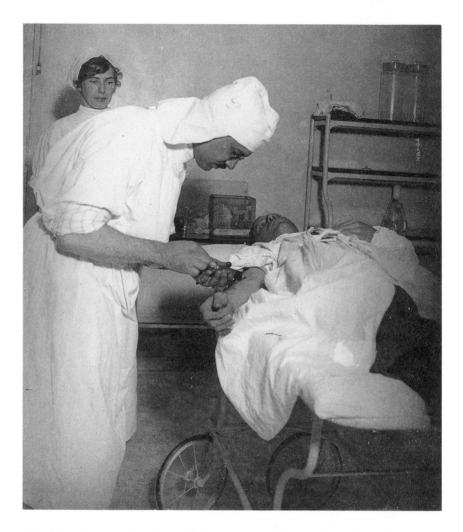

Fig. 10   Abraham Zingher withdrawing blood from a donor for polio serum,
August 1916 (Bettmann Archives)

injected into monkeys did not produce polio. Immunizing an
animal by successful vaccinations with the attenuated virus, "after the method of Pasteur," seemed to him promising.[108] Even
Emerson admitted that "in the minds of the general public and
of most physicians, there exists a close analogy between the use

of serum in epidemic meningitis and in poliomyelitis, and its success in the former has influenced them to have faith in the latter."[109]

Least critical was the popular press. Newspaper editors immediately realized that the call for blood donors could be turned into an effective publicity campaign. This campaign offered newspapers the opportunity to publish touching stories about young children offering their blood. In one case, a man with a twisted leg and limp arm supposedly told Zingher:

> I've had a tough time of it, ever since the disease left me this way as a child. . . . Vicious people [had made me] the butt of their fun and sensitive people have hurt me by avoiding me as if I were an unclean thing. All my life I've felt that I had no place in the world, that I was left out of everything worthwhile—until today. Now . . . I am happy because you tell me that I may be able to save some other human being from my fate. If I can do that I shall feel that I have not been wasted in this life.[110]

The blood serum campaign offered some members of the public an active role in attempts to prevent and treat polio, beyond swatting flies or disinfecting humans. After reading about these campaigns, Frederick H., another New Yorker, wrote to Flexner offering blood from his son who had had the disease ten years before. His son, the man boasted, had recovered so well that he "is now somewhat of an athlete."[111]

The public response suggests that the serum was believed more than just a therapy: it was seen as a cure. In 1910 a "most anxious mother" from Michigan wrote to Flexner enclosing a clipping on polio from the *Chicago Tribune*, asking whether the article's optimistic tone was accurate. Her two-year-old son had had the disease, and his right leg was helpless. "Will you please suggest a course of treatment or give me prices of what it would cost me to bring him to you," she wrote. "I have very little means but could I not work some, & earn part of our expenses. I will do anything & part with my last cent to procure help for our only little boy."[112] Similarly, a Connecticut man with a sick one-year-old baby asked Flexner whether it was true that "you have discovered a serum w[h]ich cures" the disease. "Kindly advise me what you can do in regard to same sicknes[s]," he wrote, "as I have tri[e]d so many doctors for the past four weacks [sic] and no ones seames [sic] to [k]now anything about the cure."[113]

Not all physicians and lay citizens were convinced. Some doctors warned against laboratory scientists who uncritically promoted the tools of scientific medicine. Edmond Melville, a New York physician, scornfully compared such techniques to those used by an older medical generation: "Procuring samples of blood or stomach contents, the injection of serums and vaccines and the reactions from such injections are very distasteful to most patients, more especially if they have recovered from a similar illness under the old regime."[114] Lay men and women remained similarly suspicious. In 1915 some members of the public blamed a polio outbreak on smallpox vaccination, a reaction reflecting a long-standing anti-vaccination movement.[115]

In denouncing the serum, some practitioners refused to accept the authority and assurances of scientific experts. Eugene Barton, a Pennsylvania chiropractor, warned: "First it is vaccination for typhoid fever, anti-toxin for diphtheria, now normal blood serum for Infantile Paralysis, what next?" How, Barton wondered, did Zingher or any other physicians know whether the serum worked?

> If you will take notice they claim they are not positive. It is just a hit or miss with them and very often the latter. . . . It seems as though the people of this century were unable to think and reason for themselves, but leave it all for the medical profession. As long as the people are so blind and fail to use the proper amount of reason and intelligence and to think for themselves, just so long will the medical profession pull the wool over the eyes of the public.[116]

It was difficult, perhaps impossible, for contemporaries to assess the efficacy of serum therapy for polio. When used to prevent the appearance or lessen the severity of paralysis it often seemed successful. But many untreated polio patients also experienced only mild paralysis and sometimes none at all. When the serum was used as a preventive measure, investigators found it hard to eliminate sanitary and environmental factors in determining the serum's relative success. This uncertainty apparently did not lessen the serum's popularity; perhaps it even added to its appeal. Serotherapy seemed at least as effective as instructional leaflets, fly screens, or disinfectants, and it could be legitimated as scientific through its link to immunological research and such eminent names as Emil Behring and Louis Pasteur.

Spinal fluid analysis and polio serotherapy were clearly a part of the new armamentarium of scientific medicine introduced in the early twentieth century. Their use involved the tools and techniques of laboratory science: culture media, a microscope, sometimes a centrifuge. For further study it was necessary to have experimental animals (and monkeys were expensive), complicated laboratory equipment, adequate time for research, and access to a substantial amount of clinical material.

Hospital clinicians and pathologists were mostly enthusiastic about the serum and spinal fluid analysis because these techniques reinforced the importance of the laboratory and specialized skills. Public health officials also welcomed tools to enable them to obtain rapid and unambiguous results; thus, they could feel confident in their ability to identify and isolate polio patients. Officials incorporated these new tools into health department routines, without giving up traditional sanitary and educational measures, but remained cautious by not promising the public too much.

The techniques were not, however, accepted by all physicians and patients. To some doctors, the use of these techniques reinforced the separation of the private physician from the laboratory investigator. Members of the public criticized excessive faith in laboratory solutions over experiential knowledge and more traditional methods of diagnosis and therapy.

These critiques were strengthened by the knowledge that during this period diagnostic and therapeutic techniques were often uncertain and ambiguous. The laboratory offered polio researchers various techniques and materials for experimentation, but it had limited means to solve polio's problems of transmission, prognosis, or therapy. Lumbar puncture, for example, was best employed by a specialist, and a diagnosis of polio was often followed simply by the prescription: isolation and bedrest.

Nor did the use of spinal fluid analysis and serotherapy necessarily undermine traditional ideas of the workings of disease. The tools were based on the new sciences of bacteriology and immunology, but doctors using them continued to hold theories based on humors, body imbalance, disinfection, and shifting disease etiology. Although at the Rockefeller Institute in New York, the "germ" of polio caused only polio, not tonsillitis or any other disease, in Minnesota some local physicians maintained a flexible concept of disease and rejected the notion of disease specificity.

Certainly, the laboratory contributed to a systematic approach to the study of polio. But, at the same time, its integration into clinical practice took away power from the individual physician and patient. Now, the clinician's naked eye was no longer as reliable or useful in diagnosis. Even laymen could identify "infantile paralysis," but was that the defining sign of acute anterior poliomyelitis? Forcing a patient to undergo an intrusive procedure whose products were difficult to interpret implied a new kind of medicine and a new role for the pathologist. Employing a serum exacerbated the distinction between specialist and general practitioners.

Although health officials continued to stress the importance of environmental conditions in shaping the nature of this disease, the broad environment became virtually invisible in most diagnostic and therapeutic investigations by staffs at the Rockefeller Institute, city hospitals, and other research institutions. This narrower emphasis on germs and body products did not mean that the disease had become objectively "scientific." Private physicians continued to select and interpret their diagnostic and therapeutic technologies in the context of patients and their families. Both defensive and optimistic as they debated how to bring the laboratory closer to bedside medicine, private practitioners embraced and critiqued the methods and authority of science. With the promise of scientific precision came the specter of the pathologist and clinical specialist under the shadow of the laboratory.

CHAPTER FOUR

Written in Haste: Polio and the Public

In August 1916 Mrs. C. M., a doctor's widow from Jersey City, New Jersey, wrote to the head of the Rockefeller Foundation. She had heard that the Foundation had already spent fifty thousand dollars to fight the polio epidemic, but to no avail; cases and deaths were being reported every day. Scientists' experiments using animal extracts, she explained, had "no curative qualities" and were based on "uncertain theories." She asked for financial help, but not for "research" purposes as she already had the cure for polio in a formula from her late husband's collection. There were only a few bottles left, so she needed the money to have "experts" make up the formula in large quantities to be able to wipe out the "fearful epidemic." Hers was no "empty theory" for she was already treating a "stricken patient." She reminded the Foundation that the epidemic's quarantine restrictions were causing much inconvenience to the public and to business. Signing her letter "in haste" she awaited a reply.[1]

Polio epidemics and the widespread publicity they attracted spurred a number of lay men and women to ponder the nature of the disease. They offered their families and neighbors advice and treatment, tried to sell cures, and debated the cause of these epidemics. Their responses to the actions of health officials and research scientists whose work was reported in daily newspapers suggest a popular awareness of the major medical crises of the day: the problems of polio diagnosis and therapy; its puzzling epidemiology; and the tension in public health work between dirt and germs.

The popular press reported that even the most eminent laboratory scientists could neither explain polio's origin and transmission nor predict its spread. Physicians did not know how to cure the disease and argued about the relative merits of diagnostic and therapeutic measures. Some lay Americans took these admissions of ignorance and confusion as calls for action. "According to the papers," mused Mrs. L. B. of Otego, New York, "one theory seems to be as good as another."[2] Any person, they reasoned, whether medically trained or not, could suggest a cause and cure for polio, with an eye to both helping humanity and financially benefiting themselves.

During the 1916 epidemic, members of the public, expressing concern and offering explanations, wrote to experts. More than two hundred of their letters survive, and they form the basis of this chapter. These writers were eager to discuss their ideas with those they identified as the most prominent figures associated with the epidemic: Simon Flexner, director of the Rockefeller Institute laboratories, widely quoted in the popular press; his patron John D. Rockefeller, whose Foundation organized conferences during the 1916 epidemic and provided funds for the study of the disease (but not, as many assumed, to reward the finder of a cure); John P. Mitchel, mayor of New York City, the center of the 1916 epidemic; and Mitchel's Health Commissioner Haven Emerson.

The sick, historians have reminded us, "constitute important objects of historical study."[3] Medicine is a dynamic process of negotiation between doctor and patient within the context of family and community. In the last two decades medical historians, increasingly influenced by social history, have sought the testimony of ordinary men and women. Historians have begun to explore the important roles that patients and their families have played in the development of American medical culture by examining the ways health and illness have been understood by the lay public.

Until recently there has been surprisingly little interest in the lay public in the twentieth century. Historians have more often studied lay experiences with illness in the seventeenth, eighteenth, and nineteenth centuries.[4] The limited historical attention to the patient's perspective in the recent past is paradoxical, given that lavished on other aspects of this period, such as U.S. medical education and the medical profession. Rima Apple and Judith Walzer Leavitt, however, in studies of infant feeding and childbirth have integrated the insights of women's history through their presentation of women making their own medical experience and choosing among the options offered by grandmothers and doctors.[5] My study of polio and the public is not presented from the *patient's* perspective, for most polio patients before 1920 were not yet five years old. Historians who study the health and illness of very young children may need to fashion new ways to study relations between these important "objects" and their healers. But this chapter does offer a *lay* perspective: the view of patients' parents, their neighbors, and other observers who responded to the fearful epidemics of the 1910s. Their letters, directed to public figures, framed in a public voice, do not necessarily represent what was debated privately among family and friends. In emphasizing ideas rather than experience, this chapter should be read in conjunction with my earlier discussion of the relations between officials and the lay public.

Most of these letters were not taken seriously by the experts who received them. The letters that now fill file folders in Simon Flexner's papers are categorized under "Crank Letters and Fantastic Theories." Flexner rarely answered them, but occasionally urged a correspondent to contact an orthodox physician or read his most recent piece on polio in a medical journal. Writers themselves were conscious that their suggestions were among the many. "I want to join the multitudes of fools who make suggestions in the matter of infantile paralysis," one man began his letter.[6] Haven Emerson devoted a few pages in his monograph on the 1916 epidemic to the letters his department had received; he commented that "one hardly knows whether to laugh at the fantasies or weep over the ignorance and superstition exhibited."[7]

As historians we need do neither. We should be prepared to take seriously these authors' beliefs and alternative explanations as at the same time we identify their fantastical side. These letters demonstrate to the historian, if not to the contemporary scientist, some plausible interpretations of the management of illness, a familiarity with some aspects of the theory and practice of medical science, and a striking faith in the scientific method. Their letters suggest that the meanings of science were diffuse and ambiguous. In their responses to epidemic polio, members of the public were no less entranced, reflective, and confused than contemporary scientists, health officials, and private physicians. As we have seen, many physicians and health officials were uncomfortable with certain aspects of scientific medicine: its tendency to reduce disease to an etiological agent; the shift in public health work from the environment to the individual; the increasing turn from clinician to laboratory technician. But what stands out most clearly is that most writers sought the stamp of science and tried to integrate the new theories of germs, laboratory methodology, and definitions of medical orthodoxy and authority into their own ideas.

Nonetheless, lay commentators did not hesitate to criticize the theories and practice of contemporary scientists and orthodox physicians. Although their letters demonstrate a popular interest in laboratory science and its products and a knowledge of germs, injections, culture medium, the microscope, and the test tube, their various explanations of health and disease may be described as an ecological critique. This view was consciously distinct from what they saw as the etiological reductionism of the new sciences. Although they accepted that science could play a role in healing and preventing disease, their theories and practices moved beyond the laboratory. This approach stemmed, in part, from a sense of the importance of understanding the dangers of their own environment in order to protect homes and families from disease. Their letters demonstrate a complex, contradictory, and fragmented understanding of scientific medicine and suggest rapid if selective diffusion of the new sciences of bacteriology and immunology.

The management of polio epidemics by American health officials in the early twentieth century had to some extent reinforced the idea that ordinary individuals had a potent role to play, that their cooperation was vital in preventing the spread of the disease. The mayors of New York City, Philadelphia, and Newark urged citizens to keep themselves and their city clean, report suspicious cases to the health department, respect quarantine regulations, and be ready to send affected children to city hospitals for observation and treatment. Private physicians argued that the most effective therapy would be applied if parents recognized the mild and fleeting early signs of the disease.

Scientists at the Rockefeller Institute and consulting physicians in city and private hospitals, however, looked instead toward laboratory-based solutions in which the patient's and community's participation played a minor role. The research agenda pursued by Flexner, as we have seen, emphasized virological investigation. Rockefeller scientists believed that the disease would be controlled as they came to understand more about the nature of the virus and paid little attention to its clinical or epidemiological features. But this search proved frustrating in polio therapy, diagnosis, and epidemiology. According to one Rockefeller scientist, many members of the public "looked on the Institute as the home of miracle workers," but some lay writers were skeptical of the merits of this reductionist approach.[8] Did finding a "germ," they wondered, help to either explain or understand polio?

THE WRITERS

Although epidemic polio in 1916 attacked mainly urban industrial centers in the Northeast, citizens from as far away as Canada and Texas sent advice to New York officials.[9] These writers argued that professionals trained in science or based at a scientific institution were not necessarily the most capable of controlling this disease. Many wrote as "philosophers" and experimenters themselves. Some mentioned formal training in medicine or science; most admitted only to a "medical turn of mind." A number of women had gained their expertise as a result of experience with family and neighborhood illnesses, and there were men engaged in businesses that gave them the opportunity to ponder their society's health problems.

The racial and ethnic background of those who wrote to experts during 1916 cannot be definitely identified, and their gender was roughly equally divided. Women wrote frequently as domestic healers. Homemakers and mothers urged officials to take their experience as seriously as that of a professional scientist or physician. Leila M. of Los Angeles, who suggested that the germs of adults with colds could be passed on to children and cause the more deadly paralytic disease, added "this is simply women's intuition, I may be wrong, I may be right. . . . Imagination will do no harm, and sometimes accomplishes wonders."[10] Many other women mentioned their place in the domestic sphere: mother, aunt, grandmother, or neighbor. A few called themselves nurses, some by virtue of professional training and others by virtue of caring for relatives and neighbors. Their letters demonstrated a confidence from their experience as healers and a knowledge of the results of other medicines. Mrs. A. W., a "graduate trained nurse" from Hartford, Alabama, promised that "I Can Cure Infantile Paralysis [cases] if I can be with them when first taken I Can Cure them at once and leave no bad after Effect."[11]

Men referred to their occupation to give some experiential authority to their idea. An ironworker from Youngstown, Ohio, discovered that the fumes he worked with were health-giving and suggested that victims of polio be given similar gases to inhale. Caesar R., working in a hotel on Fifth Avenue in New York City as a "wine cellar man," asked Flexner to come and discuss his theory there. Samuel K., a Jewish food merchant from Brooklyn, suggested that, if freezing the polio germ could kill it, victims should be placed in refrigerated boxes, similar to those in which fruit and meat were stored. He was "no physician," he told Flexner, admitting that his proposal might "sound ridiculous to suggest to such learned men."[12]

With an eye to possible financial rewards from the Rockefeller
Foundation, writers who did mention their economic standing
frequently pleaded poverty. Most were careful, though, to distinguish between a discoverer's just reward and charity. One
woman described her family's financial plight. With "fate
against us in every way," she and her husband had "come to the
point in life where we do not know which way to turn and about
given up all hope." But, she hoped that her polio remedy would
cure humanity and be her salvation as well, for "we are good
refined people, and deserving." She volunteered herself to the
Rockefeller Institute if the scientists there wished to test her
remedy further.[13] Another asked, after discussing his idea,
whether Flexner could use an apprentice in his laboratory "to
wash test[-]tubes."[14] A few used the occasion to ask for additional help. A New Jersey man not only wanted Flexner to test
his polio cure but also requested old leather gloves, pants, and a
suit. Financial troubles, he explained, had left him able to afford
neither the ingredients to his medicine nor the "salve for my
ulcer sores nor ointment for Eczema."[15]

About one-third of these letters asked for money outright,
although most couched their request in hesitant language.
"Some tell me to ask a million," one writer reflected. "Others
say that I am not a good citizen to ask anything."[16] Some writers
were clearly quacks, seeking to exploit the public fear of polio
for profit. The hope of financial reward had been boosted by
reports in local newspapers about the Rockefeller Foundation's
grant of $50,000 "to fight infantile paralysis," and by congress-
men who suggested that the federal government offer a gold
medal and $100,000 to the discoverer of a polio preventative or
cure.[17] But in addition to a reward, citizens hoped that a scientist or public official would take their ideas seriously. They were
not satisfied with just suggesting a cure; they wanted Flexner
and other Rockefeller scientists to test it and report back. A
handful were concerned that their names should not be made
public; others, worried that their discoveries would be overlooked, sought publicity. "Do not loose [sic] any time if you want
to know the real cause," Orville M. K. warned John D. Rockefeller, "no-one can give you the real cause better than I can . . .

[and] If I was not a poor man caused by a big loss of prosperity I would gladly give [you] this discovery for nothing."[18]

THE AUTHORITY OF SCIENCE AND THE EXPERT

Domestic remedies were clearly familiar to many of these writers. The extent of knowledge of herbs and chemicals suggests that many families cared for sick members at home, without calling in a professional physician. Their familiarity with drugs horrified Haven Emerson. Referring to recent restrictions against the prescription of medicine by unlicensed practitioners, he warned against "a lifetime of illegal practice upon a too gullible public" and cautioned the public not be "deceived" by patent medical cures.[19] Yet domestic healers, seeing themselves as expert and knowledgeable as orthodox physicians, were clearly seen as experts by others. After successfully treating their own families, some writers were asked by neighbors to treat other patients and were usually eager to do so. Hugh B. W., a clerk on the Queensland Railways in northern Australia, "knowing that medical men had failed to effect cures [of polio]," successfully treated first his daughter and then "three other cases."[20]

The domestic healers, who based their knowledge on empirical observation and experience, were nonetheless aware of the new laboratory sciences. Many recognized that their remedies and reasoning did not sound scientific or up-to-date. But they stressed that scientists such as Flexner should learn to value the traditional and the old-fashioned. A Nashville nurse reminded Flexner of the efficacy of fresh beefsteak, "an Old Time remedy which our Grandmothers resorted to in several cases of fever." Empirical results could be sufficient legitimation; at least "see the results for yourself," one man urged Flexner.[21]

They saw their work as domestic healers complementary to and frequently better than orthodox medicine. Both Mrs. C. M., the doctor's widow from Jersey City, and her husband's patients accepted that medical "formulas" (which seemed to have been strongly identified as the late doctor's property) could be selected and given by lay healers. Mrs. C. M. appeared less sure of her ability to continue her husband's work of preparing remedies from written prescriptions, but other writers were more confident. Mrs. Addie S. offered "a mother's idea": polio therapy that included baths, massage, blackberry brandy, castor oil, and enemas. She had treated a paralyzed child with this method, and the attending physician had assured her, she claimed, that without her treatment the boy would have died. Mrs. Addie S. was sure that if any of her own five children developed polio, "I'd use this same treatment in addition to the doctor's drugs."[22] Mothers in Newark, New Jersey, tied camphor balls around their children's necks during the 1916 epidemic, reflecting a long-standing folk belief that certain smells would drive away disease.[23]

Despite confidence in their own expertise many writers did turn to orthodox physicians, consulting as many as three or four.[24] Edward O. of Irvington, New Jersey, who described himself as neither doctor nor scientist but "a common half-crippled layman," sent a one-ounce bottle of polio "Antiseptic" to an Irish doctor in Newark. The Newark physician replied that "almost every mail brings up samples of just this sort with recommendations that almost tempt us to use them." But Edward O. believed that the doctor's refusal stemmed from prejudice against Germans such as himself and decided to turn to a German doctor rather than an Irishman.[25] Occasionally discoverers claimed that their family physician had urged them to ask scientists at the Rockefeller Institute to test their remedies.[26] Patients also promoted the remedies of their physicians. Katherine T. of Kansas City urged Rockefeller to contact a "wonderful" English doctor who, as the guest of a local Kansas physician, had cured patients not only of polio but also consumption and "bright disease." "Of course," she added, "he does not know that I am writing this."[27]

Writers turned to relatives and neighbors when they became dissatisfied with orthodox care. During the 1916 epidemic Mrs. Frances B. from Chicago wrote to Simon Flexner about her niece. The girl had been sick some years before, and the aunt now compared her symptoms to Flexner's descriptions of polio reported in her local newspaper. All her life, she told him, she had been of a "medical turn of mind," so she had tried to treat her niece's illness, although she was not a doctor. A trained physician, whose patient the niece had been, had left the case "offended" because he would not share a patient. The aunt reminded Flexner that fourteen years earlier she had written to him about her theory of hookworm disease and had received no reply. Did he think her niece had polio, and that her experience with the disease might benefit others fighting it now?[28]

This woman's letter suggests that physicians could be useful in managing illness, but they were ambiguous figures. Lay men and women expected conflicts not only about divergent therapies but also from offended professional pride. Mrs. Frances B. was not surprised that her niece's doctor had left the case; in fact, she may have expected, perhaps wanted, him to leave. After all, she had become the child's principal healer. One writer noted sardonically that, after giving doctors thousands of dollars to try to cure his child of tuberculosis, he had cured her and sixteen others himself, while "her doctor sleeps in his grave of consumption."[29] Similarly, scientists' approval was both sought and criticized. The Jersey City widow distrusted experiments with monkeys and scientific theorizing, but she wanted experts to make up her husband's formula. Other writers directly contacted scientists at the Rockefeller Institute; they sought approval of their discoveries and pleaded with Flexner to let his researchers test their remedies.

These healers were not necessarily altruistic; nor did they share the idea that scientific knowledge should be available for all. Indeed at times they presented themselves as medical entrepreneurs. Captain John T. of Trenton, New Jersey, consulted a man, "not a doctor," about his paralyzed brother and then instructed his mother to mix together certain oils and fats to make a salve. Three days later the brother was walking again, even though three doctors had said the case was hopeless. This writer offered the salve prescription to Flexner "providing I get something out of it." Captain John T.'s family may have shared his attitude to healing, for he reported that after his brother's cure his mother refused to give the salve to the three doctors or anyone else.[30]

To convince their eminent readers that they were neither crazy people nor quacks, some writers referred to their own training in medicine and science. A "Discoverer" from San Francisco had, he claimed, studied medicine and attained "some experience" with pathology, although he had not yet secured "a certificate." Many stressed that they took their knowledge of science and its methods seriously. A Newark woman, whose father had successfully treated tetanus and pneumonia with tincture of lobelia, added that "Pa was no mere novice nor trifler."[31] Lobelia, the central drug of the botanic Thomsonian sect of the early nineteenth century, clearly had some remaining adherents.[32]

Even those who extolled the virtues of domestic medicine expressed a faith in the values and methods of medical science. "You have the power to prove it as I as have proved it here," one man told Flexner, while urging the scientist to test his remedy by inoculating monkeys at the Rockefeller laboratories with a special curative oil. This oil was "a plain simple homemade preparation but is the highest perfection in curative science," he assured Flexner and offered to come to New York to assist in the experiments if he were given funds for travel expenses, for "I would like to work with you."[33] Another writer was concerned about the bad reputation that laboratory scientists were receiving from the popular press. The Anti-Compulsory Vaccination Society, he noted, had printed a notice in a Newark newspaper stating that it had been "clearly proven that vaccination is the cause of infantile paralysis." Make a "thorough investigation and report the facts," he urged Flexner, for it was "very disturbing to read such news, especially at this time." To explain his interest, he added that he was "a believer in Materia Medica and also a father."[34]

Others, too, showed a confidence in the tools of the laboratory. Mrs. Emma S. of Brooklyn urged scientists to make a microscopic examination of bedbugs to look for the germs of infantile paralysis.[35] Such statements reflected the belief that scientists had valuable technological resources not available to ordinary citizens. During the 1916 epidemic the manager of one company wrote to scientists at the Rockefeller Institute requesting their opinions of his company's "Nu Polish." "We do not want an analysis," he assured his audience, "all we want to know is will the finished product as it stands kill the germ causing the infantile paralysis?" He hoped that his product would prevent the polio germ "from being flipped from place to place in the house while the housewife is doing her dusting."[36]

Writers sought to apply both the methods and ideas of contemporary science. The germ theory of disease appeared in somewhat singular forms. May W., a schoolteacher from the Midwest, had seen, she claimed, many cases of infantile paralysis. The afflicted child, she had noted, always had a parent who worked with horses, and she wondered whether the polio germ might develop in horses and then be transmitted to children. She urged Flexner to test this theory with "proper blood tests and scientific research."[37] Other writers drew analogies between the laboratory and the bedside. If oxygen could interfere with the "growth of anaerobic organisms," reasoned one man from Houston, Texas, perhaps it could be tried as therapy as well.[38]

A few remedies echoed the experiments made by health officials in developing a polio serum; the use of the blood of frogs, horses, and humans appealed to some. A Brooklyn man who expressed his faith in both disinfectants and the laboratory suggested that scientists try injecting the water from jars of leeches as a possible preventive therapy.[39] Fanny M. wondered whether a serum could not "be made of mosquitoes and experimented with, on animals?" She hoped her idea might suggest "some other theory to some other superior mind."[40]

After Flexner had shown that the virus appeared in nose and throat secretions, there were numerous suggestions about disinfection.[41] One woman proposed intraspinal injections of human saliva, perhaps as a form of vaccination. A Philadelphia man claimed to have been using a nose and throat disinfectant for over twenty-five years against infections. He had used it during diphtheria epidemics before the "days of antitoxin," and in

1916 his family—all seven children—used it daily during the polio epidemic.[42]

Despite their reliance on science and its methods, some members of the public criticized its institutions and practitioners. Scientists, writers complained, were unwilling to try anything new. An agent of a Virginia chemical company, who had tried unsuccessfully to see Mitchel and Emerson during the 1916 epidemic, asked whether the city's health department was testing only things recommended "by some Doctor of high standing or the medical journals." "They do not know it all," he pointed out, "as it shoews [sic] in the results they are having."[43]

Why, lay writers asked, were scientists not open to alternatives, if, as many writers assumed, science and the search for truth in nature was democratic? A few writers, identified with unorthodox medical sects, complained that the Rockefeller Institute was interested only in testing therapies from regular physicians. One man was outraged that sectarian practitioners were not treated with respect. Years earlier, he recalled, a chiropractor, who had offered his "services and time" to the Institute to help cure polio, had received "the curt reply 'Nothing doing,' " signed by an eminent physician. An Australian lay hydropath suggested that the Institute entrust a few polio patients to the care of a good hydrotherapist. He himself had cured his own child and others with this method. "These are absolute facts," he explained, "and though I am a layman I have [been] studying physiology[,] pathology &c for some years." The tone of his letter, however, implied that he did not believe that water therapy would be taken seriously by Rockefeller scientists.[44]

During the 1910s, as scientists and physicians remained unable to treat polio or predict its spread, members of the public continued to argue that lay ideas were insightful and important. Some apologized for their temerity but argued that even highly trained professionals might occasionally benefit from lay ideas, however unlikely or outrageous. Mrs. L. B., "like most mothers," had been "much concerned and interested in the search for the cause of infantile paralysis." She urged that "however childish" her ideas about polio being spread by infected milk and beef might appear "to the scientific mind," the cause of the epidemic "was still an open question where even a busy house-wife may be privileged to express her self in a simple idea." Another woman had written to her local papers, but none would publish her letters. She contacted two doctors, "but they all laugh at me & as much as call me crazy." "I have only a simple education," she admitted, "but my mind is as sound as my body."[45] Despite lack of formal medical training, many writers urged officials to give their ideas a fair hearing. "I am a Poor Man Only an Oil Salesman" wrote another, "but I have my ideas."[46]

POLIO THERAPIES

In explaining their remedies many writers had definite ideas about how the body worked and how it could be healed. They called diseases by both technical and popular names: tuberculosis and consumption, pneumonia and grippe, polio and infantile paralysis. They also identified those illnesses, a surprisingly extensive list, which they argued could be handled by a lay healer. Their knowledge of the ingredients shows that many therapies were part of a family's domestic repertoire.

Nor did these healers use only mild botanical therapies. Their ingredients included both herbal items and chemicals and other nonnatural drugs. A frequent emphasis on remedies as "simple" and "homemade" suggests a suspicion of compound therapies, but writers used mixed ingredients as well. Their letters also indicate that it was not difficult to obtain many potent drugs in an era where most drug prescriptions were renewable at the action of patient and druggist. One "perfectly harmless" remedy had ingredients "from the Drug Store," a writer explained.[47]

Household materials were popular. A Canadian man, explaining that "this is no diagnostic but it counteracts the germ," enclosed a small brown packet of dried leaves and berries.[48] Some writers assumed that their scientific audience would know how to make herbal teas and salves; others felt it necessary to explain the preparations.

In addition to herbal therapies, familiar domestic items

included alcohol, coffee beans, potato broth, water, and salt. Haven Emerson listed more than one hundred internal remedies from letters sent to his department, including table salt and the "free use" of rum, champagne, and brandy.[49] Among the chemical ingredients were sodium chloride, kerosene, iodine, the new drug salvarsan (an arsenic compound) and its cousin mercury, black gunpowder, and the disinfectants urotropin and hydrogen peroxide, which, as we have seen, were also recommended by regular physicians. Mrs. M. R. believed that hydrogen peroxide could cure not only polio and consumption but also "nearly all of the Suffering of humanity."[50] Like experienced cooks, however, these domestic healers rarely specified exact amounts.

These healers expected predictable, visible results from their therapies. As Charles Rosenberg has shown, both patients and physicians in nineteenth-century America judged the efficacy of a therapy by the distinct physical changes it produced in a patient's body. These writers similarly stressed the importance of increasing sweating, vomiting, or excretion. Even bloodletting remained popular.[51] These physiological changes were a sign to both healer and patient of the extent of the sickness, the efficacy of the treatment, and the progress of the disease.[52]

The public dissatisfaction with regular polio therapies may have reinforced this emphasis on drugs and therapies that produced such definite physiological effects. The laboratory had provided few specific therapies for polio, and scientists seemed to stress accurate diagnosis over treatment. These healers confidently mixed the old with the new. A Brooklyn woman who had been using "large doses" of quinine since the start of the 1916 epidemic felt that domestic remedies should be combined with scientific techniques. "Make a lumbar puncture if you will," she told Flexner, "but don't wait to hear from it before beginning treatment."[53]

In these letters polio was defined symptomatically, a notion reinforced by a frequent use of the popular term "infantile paralysis." Orthodox physicians, as we have seen, were unsure that the classification "poliomyelitis" properly described the disease and had frequently designated it a "general infection."

Polio's symptoms, certainly, were not distinctive until the final stages of paralysis. Both lay healers and professional physicians also remained uneasy about the concept of etiologic specificity; they still saw diseases shift from mild to more serious. "There is a marked paralellism [sic] between Infantile Paralysis and La Grippe," Eugene G. of Denver wrote, for polio "may act like a chamaelion [sic] and change face as it progresses."[54]

Most therapies proposed in these letters focused exclusively on the clinical symptoms of polio and were intended to cool fever, dull pain, strengthen blood and nerves, and restore function to paralyzed limbs. Heat therapy was popular, applied in baths, bandages, and as steam. Writers also discussed techniques for massaging paralyzed limbs and homemade or patent electricity kits to help invigorate deadened nerves.

These techniques were cheap, relatively simple to employ, and chosen with an eye to other domestic healers. "A "Washingtonian" told scientists at the Rockefeller Institute that capsules made of quinine, jalap, and black pepper were completely effective and could be administered "easily by any reputable person."[55] Thirty-nine (around 15 percent) of Emerson's correspondents proposed poultices, blisters, liniments, and healing oils—therapies that not only reflected those employed by regular physicians but also those nonprofessional healers could use when trained physicians were unavailable or too expensive. A woman from Tioga County, New York, described her massage and bathing treatment in detail; then she added that "any mother can do as I did."[56]

The success of these therapies was judged by empirical observation of their effects, on not only others but also their discoverer. A Florida man had made himself "immune to yellow fever" after twenty-five years of experiments and was now sure that his remedy (bismuth and oil of winter green) could also cure polio. Mrs. W. H. of Butte, Montana, who had suffered for some years from pain and "melancholia," had started to experiment on herself and "in desperation took internally a germicide" after her doctor told her that he could no longer help her. This, she was sure, would also cure paralysis. She assured Flexner that she was "not some quack woman" but "worthy of your consideration."[57]

If a disinfectant countered pain and depression, then it might also temper fever and paralysis. Mrs. W. H. and others like her did not feel that their therapies had to be specific to one symptom or disease. A Pittsburgh man suggested trying "intraspinal" injections of either salvarsan or mercury; he was sure that their potent effect in the treatment of venereal disease would make them equally efficacious for paralysis. Sarah S. from Rochester, New York, believed her remedy would cure not only polio but also goiter, catarrh, extreme running sores, stomach trouble, and blood poisoning. It was, she claimed, "entirely anticeptic [sic]" and both a disinfectant and a deodorizer; that is, it attacked disease in both body and air.[58] Louise M. of New York City compared polio to diphtheria, after an undertaker told her about a child who had died of polio that "he was positive that dip[h]theria was present in a most decided form, because the body takes exactly the same amount of embalming fluid that a dip[h]theria case takes." The undertaker, she stressed, was "very sincere in his views."[59]

If these writers demonstrated a continuing belief in domestic empiricism, attacked abstract scientific theorizing, and remained skeptical of etiological specificity, many also showed a popular interest in the germ theory. They used terms such as germs, microbes, organisms, and phagocytes.[60] The term germs was used interchangeably with "animals" and "parasites" so one remedy had "intense bacteriotropic, antitoxic and spoliating and anti-thermal power."[61] And germs were often the source of not one disease but many.[62]

Writers were inspired by the efficacy of techniques based on the new sciences of bacteriology and immunology. The 1916 epidemic reminded one writer of a child who some years before had developed polio and diphtheria, was given antitoxin, and recovered from both diseases. Could the diphtheria germ or its antitoxin have cured the paralysis, she wondered, "or was it just one of those things that cannot be explained?" Test this idea, she urged Rockefeller scientists, for you have "everything with which to experiment."[63] Others drew from the model of bacteriology the importance of controlling disease by killing germs. If a patient's body was rubbed with kerosene oil, "the *germs* that cause infantile paralysis cannot possibly live in the presence of *kerosene oil* or its gas," promised Archibald S. of Milwaukee, Wisconsin. A few demonstrated a greater knowledge of immunology: some germs fought others, and their actions in one part of the body could be transferred to another. One man, "frankly confessing my utter ignorance of bacteriology," nonetheless argued that the "baccullis [*sic*] Buleria," which worked "beneficially" in the human intestines, would duplicate that action if injected into the spinal cord.[64]

These writers, then, were willing to make analogies between their experience and that of scientific professionals. They were confident they could judge therapy and healer. They did not see science as contradictory to domestic practice, but they frequently sought to integrate lay ideas with the methods of the new sciences. Such methods, however, were at best partially understood, and much of their incomplete knowledge the result of cursory explanations in the popular press.

THE CAUSES OF POLIO

While these men and women hoped that their domestic medicines would cure polio and arrest epidemics, many went further and offered their explanations of polio's underlying cause. They sought to explain why adults were rarely victims; why the disease appeared both in middle-class families and the poor, among both immigrants and the native-born, and increasingly in cities; and who and what spread it. Their explanations went beyond identifying the germ and its vectors; they outlined underlying contributing causes to explain how and why a particular epidemic had occurred. Explaining the causes of epidemic polio meant confronting the problems of assigning responsibility for the control of epidemic disease and identifying the proper roles of individuals, medical professionals, and health officials.

In their lifetimes these writers had seen significant physical alterations of the urban landscape. Not surprisingly, they sounded themes of disharmony and unfamiliarity, as they pondered the relation between epidemic disease and disorder in the urban environment. They sought ways to control the dangers of the city from entering their homes and threatening the health of their families.

Because polio was clearly seen as a children's disease, a major consideration was the safety of infant foods, particularly milk. Since the 1890s Progressive health reformers had engaged in fervent public debate about the relations between unsanitary milk and the high rates of urban infant mortality. Public health officials had begun to control the production and sale of milk by using the new techniques of bacteriological science to test cows and dairy farmers for tuberculosis and check milk for the "proper" level of bacteria.[65]

Pasteurization, a new method of sanitizing milk, supposedly produced a "disease-free" product but one still too expensive for many working-class families unless subsidized through a dispensary. Seeking an explanation for the appearance of polio, a writer attacked the recent "fad" of pasteurization. It was artificial, she claimed, and infants fed on this unnatural food became more susceptible to disease. Although it might prevent the transfer from farm to city of certain germs such as typhoid, measles, and scarlet fever, it also destroyed children's natural resistance to other diseases such as polio.[66]

During the 1916 epidemic Nathan Straus, a New York philanthropist who had established the first infant milk stations to provide pasteurized milk for poor mothers, acknowledged that there was public suspicion of milk as possible transmitter of the disease. He wrote angrily to Mayor Mitchel, Commissioner Emerson, and the head of the U.S. Public Health Service, asking about the recent press reports of six babies fed on Straus pasteurized milk who had contracted polio. Straus claimed to have studied twenty-five hundred children "supplied with pasteurized milk from my depots" who had "all escaped infantile paralysis." Officials, he concluded, should admit "the probability of proper pasteurization preventing such dissemination of the disease."[67]

The concept of infected milk was also a powerful epidemiological explanation, for it could explain the appearance of the disease among the rich as well as the poor. It could also resolve the problem of polio cases in homes where watchful middle-class housekeepers and mothers had guarded all forms of infection from the door. Mrs. David H. D. of Montclair, New Jersey, worried that unpasteurized milk, which was drunk by the "very poor and the rich," could be endangered by dairymen with "excreta" on their hands. Moreover, some writers were not convinced that the city's regulatory efforts had produced safe milk. As Pauline M. warned graphically, "inspectors test milk by sticking their fingers in each can and into the mouth and let it drip from the mouth into the can."[68] Mrs. Hannah G. drew Flexner a picture of a "European herb" and explained how it might have caused the epidemic by poisoning the milk of cows that had eaten it.[69]

Like health officials and private physicians, many lay citizens believed that the disease was carried from tenements to the suburbs by infected immigrants. Immigrants, whose sanitation could not be controlled, delivered a variety of services to middle-class neighborhoods, including milk, fruit, and laundry. A number of writers worried that even the most careful mother could not ensure that these items were truly safe from disease. Even though American cities were increasingly becoming racially and geographically segregated, writers worried that suburban living was not completely immune from such dangers.

Writers integrated these fears with older ideas about disease resulting from the smells and gases of filth. New York's subway system concerned many who complained about the odors, the congestion, and the mixing of classes and ethnic groups. One man suggested that the health department fumigate all subway cars, which reeked "with billions of germs, caused by the filthy foreign element constantly usenig [sic] them."[70] Writers feared that they could not control their interaction with diseased working-class and immigrant people, particulary in public arenas. Madison Square Park, for example, was seen as dangerous for "here congregate hundreds from the Congested East Side mingled at closest quarters with people from widely separated parts of our great City."[71]

In response to warnings by public health departments about the danger of poor hygiene, writers urged the use of disinfectants, including thirty-two (around 15 percent) of Emerson's correspondents. Divide the city into sections and spray them with different disinfectants and oils, suggested Mrs. B. T. The oils might help to free the air of germs.[72] Just as the New York City Department of Street Cleaning was flushing the streets of slum districts, so writers suggested disinfecting and fumigating every room in the city, subway cars, and the hands of street car conductors. During the 1916 epidemic one Virginia man was horrified to hear from a New York health official that the Health Department had discontinued disinfection as a general practice a year earlier.[73]

Writers also demonstrated a consistent concern with the domestic sphere. Housekeepers feared that the disease was entering their homes as the result of new technology. Some milk, for example, now arrived in bottles rather than being dipped out of milk cans into the waiting pails of housewives. Public officials stressed that bottled milk was cleaner and safer, but, as one writer asked, "would you like a bottle from the slums brought to your home & washed, yes, all in the one tub?"[74]

Commercial canning had begun to provide city dwellers with a wide selection of vegetables, fruits, and meats, in a form which kept food, often manufactured far from its final selling point, for long periods on store shelves. But contemporary scandals, such as the Spanish-American War's "embalmed beef" and Upton Sinclair's exposé of the meat-packing industry, had intensified fears about the dangers of filth and germs in canned and packaged foods.[75] In hot weather, one writer warned, the polio germ was activated "in some formenting [sic] or putrefying culture medium" and suggested milk and canned fish as possible culprits.[76]

Packaged and refined foods, such as bread and flour, also reminded writers of the separation of domestic economy from the production of household goods. Housewives needed to take special care and look for signs of decay or mold that might signal the development of disease germs. One writer blamed the epidemic on mold, which could be spread by mice and flies, in "bought foods," and a housewife compared packaged food with the familiarity and safety of home baked and cooked meals.[77] A "housekeeper of many years" noticed during the

1916 epidemic that breads and cereals were developing a stickiness that could herald mold, caused, she suggested, by improperly cleaned gas stoves. She suggested that families with afflicted children examine such foods carefully.[78]

There was also the potential danger of less familiar foodstuffs. As a result of improved refrigerated storage and transport systems, the expansion of national and specialized food markets, and the United States's interest in South America and other foreign lands, unusual produce such as fruits from California and Latin America had begun to appear in northern and midwestern urban markets and groceries.

Polio, writers feared, could be spread by dangerous insects such as South American tarantulas or unusual flies found inside these new foods. One woman, noticing a swarm of small insects hovering around a banana, remarked that "immediately they connected themselves in my mind with the Infantile Paralysis scourging this city." Bananas, she added, were an "abundant and popular diet here, especially among children," and "Italians deal very largely in them."[79] A sample of fruit juice developed a "foreign odor" and was tested by John K. of Jersey City. He put it in a tube for "microscopic examination" and found small flies multiplying rapidly. "Naturally I connected this with infantile paralysis," he wrote, arguing that either the juice was affected by a "rare putrifactive [sic] yeast or bacteria" or it had become infected by insects carrying "powerful patholagenic [sic] germs."[80]

Writers sought to explain why the disease appeared in many different kinds of families. A Long Island man reflected that the reason that a "healthy strong farmer" with "all new buildings" and a "high and healthy located" farm had a sick child and one who died of infantile paralysis was perhaps because cows had eaten some plant poison "since the disease attacks also well to do people, (I am thinking about cleanliness) could the disease no[t] have one common cause?"[81] Mrs. Ida S. blamed the epidemic on the seasons "when the great variety of fruits are in the hands of all classes and conditions of persons." In the sun the skin of fruits nurtured the growth of infantile paralysis germs, which had been deposited by flies and mosquitoes, she argued.

Although housewives were careful of flies, "in many cases, we bring into our homes, without thought of sterilization for lurking danger, these fruits which have been exposed to the contact with disease."[82]

Disease-carrying flies were a special concern. They could explain how polio crossed the boundaries of class, ethnicity, and hygiene. A family who lost a child to the disease was told by their doctor that it was the result of the child playing in stables among stable flies. Reflecting on this explanation, one writer agreed that a fly theory could explain why only one child in a family was attacked, why the disease appeared only on certain streets and blocks, why secluded children were safe, and why the disease traveled long distances.[83] Flies could carry disease from the sick poor to the middle-class. Germs carried by flies could spread disease from an infected dispensary patient to some other person, readers of the *Newark Evening News* were warned during the 1916 epidemic, particularly "if the individual to which it pays its attentions happens to have a scratch within reach."[84]

A concern with flies and other insects as disease carriers reflected health officials' warnings, particularly fervent during the 1916 epidemic. One writer demonstrated a knowledge of recent work in medical entomology. It was important to understand the relationship between insects and disease "in the light of science," he argued, referring to the examples of insects spreading yellow fever, malaria, sleeping sickness, and spotted fever. He suggested that polio might be spread by the black fly or buffalo gnat, for one of his horses had been paralyzed with polio by a gnat and had never fully recovered.[85]

Writers also blamed insects other than the fly. "Personally I am confident that flies, mosquitoes, lice, bed bugs, and roaches may carry to spread the disease," wrote one man.[86] Popular culprits were those insects identified with the unsanitary habits of the working class. "I have hesitated to write this letter, for fear of being [thought] absurd," explained Mrs. Jeanette L. "I trust you will understand it, and pardon me if I appear so." As a young girl she was badly "poisoned" by bed bugs, so she had a fund of knowledge about them "not common to well-bred people." Bed bugs, she suggested, could be spreading the disease as nurse maids or other servants carried them unsuspectingly into the "most carefully guarded homes" and into public places, such as plush theater seats and street-cars, and "wherever crowds gather."[87] Cockroaches, another writer pointed out, were more prevalent "among all classes of people than is generally known" due to "Ignorance, Laziness, Incompetency, and incompetent servants."[88]

These letters demonstrated fears about individuals' inability to control infection and particularly the special responsibility of the housewife and mother as guardian of the home and her family's health. Reflecting a constant theme in public health and popular literature, these writers consistently referred to the image of the home as haven in a threatening urban environment.

Manufacturers advertising household sanitary products tried to exploit the fear that disease could be carried unknowingly from the street into the house. "Fight Infantile Paralysis with Cleanliness," urged the makers of Rexall Nursery Castile soap; and the Rexall tooth paste would "Keep the Mouth Clean and Prevent Disease."[89] Whether caused by germs or insects, Fitzgerald's hair soap advertisements warned: "There is a great danger of carrying this dread disease in the hair. . . . Physicians recommend that all children's heads be washed at least twice a week."[90] Dust and dirt were seen as transmitters of disease. Scientists, readers of the *Philadelphia Inquirer* were told during the 1916 epidemic, had shown that the germs of anthrax, diphtheria, cholera, typhoid fever, and plague could enter the home on the hems of long skirts, which had been shown to carry more than a million germ "colonies." Short skirts, however, carried only about half a million and so were not only fashionable and more "appropriate for the active girl of today" but also more sanitary.[91]

The importance of cleanliness was reinforced by the tuberculosis campaigns that offered the public a powerful model of disease transmission by stressing the dangers of spitting.[92] New Public Health proponent Charles V. Chapin had also emphasized the idea that germs could be spread by the body's waste products. This emphasis was made concrete in the case of polio by Flexner's stress on nose and mouth secretions. A "Dean" from Connecticut suggested that polio was just one manifestation of tuberculosis. The spread of epidemic polio could be explained, he believed, by tubercular "afflicted persons" walking "in the gardens of the rich as well as in the alleys of the poor," scattering "dangerous sputum everywhere."[93] Polio, another writer reflected, was similar to consumption, for it was also caused by a "virus" that passed from nose and throat.[94]

That polio was a children's disease did not surprise most writers. Children were unusually vulnerable; they were unable to control the sanitation of their environment or monitor their bodies' health. Children who ate foods from outside the home risked indigestion and possible infection. Street peddlers who sold ice cream and candy were especially dangerous.[95] Writers frequently assumed that polio was the result of an unbalanced body system, whereby children lost their resistance to disease.[96] Children were particularly vulnerable when sleeping, warned one writer. "The germs can bore right into the delicate skin without meeting any resistance, thereby poisoning them, and their physical condition is not strong enough to throw off the contagion."[97]

Only with proper health education and supervision could children be protected. City children, writers warned, could pick up dried "secretions" from the swings in playgrounds or by exchanging chewing gum with seemingly healthy friends. One physician, after seeing a row of children on a park bench chewing pieces of bark, wrote to the *New York Times* urging parents to curb such bad habits, for by "exchanging pieces of the same" these children were "thereby facilitating the exchange of any infectious material."[98]

Writers also blamed poor care by parents. In one case a writer atypically accused middle-class parents of being the source of the disease. A Canadian woman blamed the epidemic on the inappropriate feeding of middle-class children. Slum mothers, she argued, had "the benefit of visiting nurses and free clinics." But wealthier children, she feared, were being fed "tidbits" from their indulgent parents' plates, thereby upsetting the digestive system and perhaps leading to dangerous infection. Furthermore, she argued, these parents were the most frequent buyers of patent medicines that were bad for the liver and the stomach. The polio germ, she suspected, was probably found in the liver. A Brooklyn writer also blamed the epidemic on bad habits, but this time smokers' nicotine was seeping into the skins of children, making them susceptible to disease.[99]

Children became vulnerable not just as the result of poor parental care and domestic dangers, but owing to the urban environment itself. City living was unnatural and especially dangerous for children, some writers argued; they suggested unusual diets to enable children to brave urban dangers. Frank F., an advertising man from Philadelphia, offered Flexner a special "life rock" that he had discovered from volcanic deposits in land he owned in Maine. It would provide the proper balance of minerals, this probable quack explained, for the epidemic was the result of children eating food and drinking water from improperly nourished soil. If children were denied crucial nutrients, they became more susceptible to disease, and a mild sickness turned into a more dramatic form. With similar reasoning, a Missouri attorney suggested that common salt might be the answer. "Years ago," he explained, "when people lived on plain coarse food, ate salt, meat, fish, and self rising breads, the disease was practically unknown." Salt, he argued, would nourish the blood and digestive organs and even be an essential germ destroyer.[100] Children needed natural not artificial food. The use of margarine was increasing as the cost of living rose, a farmer explained, but butter substitutes were dangerous for infants. "This is merely a theory with me and it may be worthless to you but I know . . . that you could not know everything about the food supply and I thought that I would get it off my mind."[101]

The idea that climate and environment played a significant role in regulating the appearance of disease was ancient. Fear about dampness, heat, and decay were reinforced by reports in the popular press.[102] A number of writers focused on changes in the weather. A man from Wilmington, Delaware, noted that the organisms of both influenza and polio were reported in medical journals to be somewhat similar, and he wondered if the influenza agent was "rendered more destructive to the brain tissue and cord, by reason of the intense heat of the summer and the unhygienic conditions existing in the largest cities." In a more bizarre explanation, Michael C. argued that the increasing ice caps and resulting negative electricity that was the "Angel of Death" were enabling germs to enter the bloodstream, causing, in addition to epidemic polio, bubonic plague in rats, hydrophobia in coyotes, homicidal mania in men, and suffragism in women.[103]

Some writers expressed dissatisfaction with health experts' lack of interest in the weather. "I am very skeptical about [the theory of] contagion," wrote one woman. Polio, she explained, was not a "Dirt Disease" but was diagnosed by a "High Class Physician" as the result of excessive "ground dampness," yet physicians were trained only in "cleanliness." Being only a lay person," she complained to Flexner, she could "do nothing to make my knowledge of benefit to humanity."[104]

These lay ideas suggest a broad concern with ecological determinants of health. Writers went beyond germs in searching for underlying causes of disorder in the physical environment that had heralded or caused the epidemics. As each epidemic "seems to be more alarming and widespread than the one preceding," one writer felt that there must be "some other contributing cause other than the germ itself."[105] A New Yorker suggested that the Health Department investigate the new buildings on his block; perhaps the digging and construction were disturbing buried germs.[106] The city environment, however, provided ample opportunity for making its citizens vulnerable to disease. Street dust, readers of the *Philadelphia Inquirer* were assured, was, next to garbage and sewage, the "most unwholesome thing" about urban life. Country dust was not as unhealthy as city dust, for it did not contain industrial fumes, such as those from chemical plants or cotton mills. But city dust could weaken the body by allowing the "insidious bacillus easy entrance."[107]

Some rejected blaming individuals and turned to environmental sources. "I wish to say emphatically that the American Italian is not to be singled out and charged with anything" other than "nationality," Ernest C. told Mayor Mitchel, angry at the blame his compatriots were receiving. He suggested the mayor consider instead the "foul sewerage odor" most noticeable in the subway between Thirty-Third and Grand Central stations, an odor which "many thousands of young and old people are obliged to endure . . . for many minutes each day."[108]

Other technological innovations were blamed, such as radio waves and electricity, both increasingly entering private and public spaces. Michael C. of San Francisco explained that "Marconni [sic] Waves and Negat[ive] Elect[ricity] evolved from the ground[,] raises temperature to fever heat" and produced "infantile paralysis, apoplexy and war madness." Having already explained the cause of polio, this writer added that he expected "fair play in competing for the $25,000."[109] A few writers suggested that the European war was at fault. Its distance from outbreaks of polio was irrelevant, for "wireless telegraphy travels to and from Germany, so distance doesn't matter." Germany, another writer explained, was depleting European and American environments of nitrogen in her wartime efforts to make gunpowder.[110]

New York City's system of garbage disposal was also criticized, particularly by Staten Island groups already battling city hall over a proposed garbage plant to be built in their borough. Blaming the epidemic on the flies accumulating around the inadequately managed city dump, they wrote regularly to the mayor of New York. "What profiteth it a City if it makes a few dollars out of garbage and slays hundred of babies?" asked the chairman of the Staten Island Civic League, who accused the mayor of "sucking a penny out of filth at the cost of babies' lives."[111]

A few observers, mainly those writing to the mayor of New York, blamed the epidemic on the urban political system. The epidemic, they argued, was a sign of the city's political corruption and the poverty and distress of its people. Benjamin M. accused Mitchel of "inexcusable cowardice in breaking your word to the people of the city and opposing the referendum on untaxing buildings." The polio epidemic was caused by "overcrowding, poor food and general poverty," he claimed, and "the bereaved parents of the children suffering from the epidemic

may properly blame you." Sometimes writers proposed solutions beyond the boundaries of Progressive reform. The "only
way you will ever prevent the wholesale slaughter of the
'kiddies' is to do away with slums, unemployment, ignorance,
starvation, and *capitalism,*" wrote a Georgia socialist, for "infantile paralysis cannot live where the workers get the full product
of their labor."[112]

Writers called on public officials and scientists for mostly secu-
lar solutions. Only a few explicitly turned to the supernatural.
Emphasizing the power of prayer may also have been an implicit attack on the religious skepticism thought characteristic of
modern scientists. "If you men of science will go down on your
knees *together* and ask the Great God of all for a cure *you will
surely find it!*" promised one writer. A New York pastor announced that it was time for "Christians of the City" to an-
nounce "our living faith in the great Physician, Jesus Christ,
who was given to the world to save it from sickness and sin when
faithfully appealed to in times of necessity like this." He urged
the mayor to "issue an urgent proclamation to the Bishops,
Pastors, and Christians of the City to unite in daily prayers—
morning, noon, and evening and continue [for] as long as necessity requires, for the relief of the afflicted children of the City."
But unlike President Zachary Taylor who, in 1849, had called
for a day of national prayer and fasting to avert cholera, Mayor
John Mitchel was silent.[113]

George B. of Chicago had been "reluctant to write" for he "had
no real faith in dreams." Although he was not a doctor, he had
read about the disease in the press and, he told Flexner, the week
before he had dreamed the cure (a combination of sea water and
electricity) "revealed to me by a scientist."[114] Believing that Flexner was "broadminded enough to consider anything which
might lead to the discovery of the cause and cure of disease even
if it does not confrom to recognized Scientific methods," Mrs. L.
L. also told him about her dream. Always considered "Psychic,"
she had recently dreamed of the human spine and heard a voice
saying, "*There is the seat of infantile paralysis.*"[115]

If orthodox medicine was associated with the civilized Chris-
tian world, unorthodox remedies were seen as the work of for-

eigners. One man was outraged at a report that scientists were testing remedies of "heathen doctors." He was probably refer- ring to a purported cure John Ly Sang and Gau F. Lee, two Chinese physicians, had offered to the New York City Depart- ment of Health in July 1916. According to the *New York Times,* they argued that polio, like a similar Chinese disease, could be cured by withdrawing the juice of a certain plant with a chicken feather and then running the feather over the afflicted parts of the patient; the juice drew the poisons to the surface. Scientists, this Montana writer remarked, should rather try prayer.[116]

In the decades after the germ theory was first explicated science played a critical and defining role in structuring debates on medical issues. To deal with the problems of epidemic polio, lay citizens turned to what they referred to as "modern science" and used its methods, authority, and vocabulary. Some also sought the public and financial support of eminent scientists and officials. Many felt that the scientific method was merely another way to demonstrate the efficacy of their remedy or explanation. With science, a new enterprise, everything seemed possible.

Whatever their opinion, most lay writers agreed that the man- agement of illness was one in which lay men and women could play a part as important as the laboratory scientist or the private physician. Writers, in fact, saw not only the concepts but also the resources of science as potentially available to anyone, to assess medical theory or treatment. With this ideal of democracy in science, they were confident that their homemade remedies deserved as rigorous and serious a test as any vaccine or serum in Flexner's Rockefeller laboratories. Some showed profound skepticism and hostility to doctors and science; some welcomed the germ theory, and others were attracted to science for merce- nary reasons. Still, in the form and structure of their letters, these men and women acknowledged the authority and pres- tige of science and scientists.

The men and women who wrote these letters stressed that they were neither quacks nor crazy. Most believed that their own experience, as city dwellers and as family and community members, enabled them to understand and explain disease and disorder in an urban environment. The northeastern city was filled with danger. To travel within it was to chance infection from objects and people whose diseased state might not be visible to the naked eye. Vision might not be trustworthy, but writers still relied on their noses to assess safety; the worse an odor the more they feared the multiplication and spread of disease.

Even the home could not provide complete safety. Health officials urged the public to insure their health through careful domestic hygiene, but some writers worried that even the domestic sphere could be endangered. Dust, germs, flies, or secretions might pass by even the most hygienically alert housekeeper. Disease could enter her doors in the form of poorly washed bottles, street dust on skirt hems, foreign fruits, or canned foods. Products such as meat and milk were delivered by immigrants whose cleanliness could not be adequately checked.

These writers' conception of the susceptibility and vulnerability to diseases that ecological hazards posed reflected some dangers of their physical environment. The manmade city held certain and potent dangers. Automobiles produced dangerous smells; factory fumes and dust from cotton mills were hazardous; open drains, faulty sewers, and filthy privies all threatened health. Locating a germ and pinpointing an infected individual, they argued, was not enough to explain or control an epidemic or ensure freedom from disease. The lay concern for environmental protection appeared just as medical experts were turning to germs and vaccines and public officials were turning away from their traditional sanitary work.

Historians must remain cautious when they consider contemporaries' use of the vocabulary of science. The use of terms such as "germs," for example, does not always indicate an acceptance among the lay of the concept as we now understand it or as laboratory scientists used it in the early twentieth century. In the early twentieth century, as the germ theory became part of a broad understanding about the workings of disease and the body, members of the public did discuss germs or "disease germs" (the qualifier is interesting). The intellectual framework for this discussion predated the nineteenth century by integrating competing traditional and new ideas of disease. Many explained the workings of disease, for example, in a miasmatic framework and worried about smells, bad air, filth, decay, and overcrowding. Similarly, their therapies were sometimes almost humoral, involving counterirritation (drawing poisons away from diseased organs), bloodletting, and numerous cathartic methods to cleanse the body. Such distinctions remind us that we need to be careful about assuming similar theoretical underpinnings in the use of scientific terms by both the lay public and contemporary physicians.

These letters add to our understanding of the popular response to early twentieth-century American urban life. These writers' knowledge of the germ theory was often sketchy and "fantastic." Yet many had a distinctive understanding of the effects of the modern industrializing city on the body, the mind, and perhaps the soul. During the 1916 epidemic citizens expressed deep-seated concerns about modern life and their changing urban environment, symbolized by the potential dangers of new buildings, streetcars, subways, canned and imported foods, and pasteurized milk. These words of men and women, written "in haste," express more clearly than in ordinary circumstances their fears about their own lives and the danger of disease.

CHAPTER FIVE

A Humble and Contrite Frame of Mind: Polio and Epidemiology

The intricacies of the polio story were worked out slowly and with difficulty during the first half of this century.[1] By the 1910s the methods and questions applied to study epidemic polio were largely established. Working within a bacteriological model, scientists had established that the germ of polio could be transmitted experimentally between laboratory animals and that, as it passed through the small pores of a filter, it was a virus rather than a bacterium. But the mechanism of the disease in nature remained unclear. Researchers were uncertain of how the virus was transmitted and how infectious it was. Rhesus monkeys used in the laboratory could only be infected by direct injection of the brain and spinal cord, and they rarely infected each other. Furthermore, laboratory animals had a higher mortality rate than humans, which suggested differing viral virulence or incomplete animal-human analogies. Rockefeller scientists found the virus in nerve cells and the spinal cord but not consistently in the bloodstream, so they emphasized polio's neurotropic nature. But if it were spread like a respiratory disease, as Simon Flexner claimed, then several questions emerged: Why were there not more cases? Why did it rarely appear more than once in a family? And why had polio become a major public health problem only since the turn of the century?

The confusion of scientists over how the disease progressed

both within the body and in the community was disturbing. European and American researchers who had established the viral etiology of polio by 1909 felt confident that etiologic precision would enable them to explain the spread of the disease and develop preventive measures. Yet this optimism had met frustrations; public health measures had neither controlled nor prevented the spread of the disease, and the available therapeutic and diagnostic tools were inadequate to treat or identify victims and carriers.

Outside the laboratory and away from the bedside epidemiological work promised clearer answers. Field researchers, trying to trace polio cases in the population, hoped to establish the cause and origin of epidemics and effective means to prevent their spread. Often in the nineteenth century such studies had proven successful. The work of American and British researchers John Snow, William Farr, and William Budd had shown that applying new statistical and investigatory techniques could explain the role played by contaminated water in spreading cholera and typhoid. This work had a strong environmentalist basis; in fact, its urban and reformist focus was an integral part of the sanitary science movement. But the germ theory threatened to undermine this explicit environmentalism. Health officials increasingly argued that bacteriological research would help them to identify infectious agents and hidden carriers, not clean up streets and sewers.[2]

When epidemic polio became a major public health problem in the early 1900s field researchers drew on both environmental and bacteriological approaches. There were numerous theories about the way the disease spread. Laboratory scientists suggested that the polio germ was spread directly from person to person through secretions from the nose and throat. The successes of medical entomology in explicating the spread of bubonic plague, sleeping sickness, yellow fever, malaria, and typhus led other researchers to stress the possibility that polio was spread by an insect or animal vector. And, despite the new emphasis on germs, some continued to explain polio's epidemiology with older theories, such as the belief that inanimate objects (fomites), dust, and other filth could spread disease.

In the early decades of the twentieth century epidemiology in America was barely a discipline. There were almost no professional epidemiologists, and the American Epidemiological Society was not founded until the 1920s.[3] Epidemiological work was usually done by medical men employed by local or state health departments, but those who studied polio also included pediatricians and general practitioners with clinical experience of the disease.

A few states became centers of epidemiological research in polio due to their extensive experience with the disease. Hibbert Winslow Hill was one of the first state-employed epidemiologists, appointed to head the Minnesota Board of Health's new division of epidemiology in 1910. Hill's reports on polio outbreaks in Minnesota during the 1900s earned him a place on the American Public Health Association's polio committee in 1911.[4] In Massachusetts officials from the State Board of Health and physicians at Harvard Medical School conducted a series of polio studies between 1907 and 1912, which tried to link epidemiological theory, clinical experience, and laboratory evidence.[5] These researchers included Milton J. Rosenau, later head of the fledgling Harvard-MIT School for Health Officers, and Robert W. Lovett, who became an eminent polio orthopedic specialist and a decade later diagnosed and treated Franklin Delano Roosevelt. The New York City Department of Health conducted epidemiological work during epidemics, and scientists who studied polio virology at the Rockefeller Institute also occasionally speculated on these topics.[6] But the most important institution employing professional epidemiologists during this period was the U.S. Public Health Service. Federal epidemiologists Wade Hampton Frost and Allen W. Freeman, who investigated New York's 1916 epidemic extensively, were both later influential teachers of the first professionally trained generation of American epidemiologists at the Johns Hopkins School of Public Health and Hygiene.[7]

When these men examined the medical literature they found that epidemic polio was a relatively new subject. There were no epidemiological studies of polio until the disease became a serious public health problem in the 1880s and 1890s.

Cases of infantile paralysis were initially the province of pediatricians and neurologists who classified polio as a rare disease affecting the nervous system of young children. Small outbreaks in the northeastern United States began to attract some broader interest. Health official Charles S. Caverly's 1894 study of 132 cases in Vermont became an early standard text in polio epidemiology.[8]

A turning point in polio epidemiology came in 1905 with the work of Swedish epidemiologist Ivar Wickman, a student of the clinician Jacob Heine who had first outlined polio's clinical features. After a careful study of outbreaks in isolated communities in rural Sweden, Wickman identified a large number of infected children without paralytic symptoms, a condition he termed "abortive." Wickman suggested that these asymptomatic cases might be hidden carriers and that polio should not be seen as solely a paralytic disease. Even though he wrote before a viral agent had been established, Wickman argued convincingly that the contagious disease was generally spread by direct contact.[9] "Until recently it has been a matter of personal opinion whether or not the disease was communicable," noted New York physician Joseph Collins in 1910, but since the publication of Wickman's work "the contagion of the disease has been admitted."[10]

But without a clear-cut diagnostic test most of Wickman's invisible cases remained unseen and uncounted. Polio cases were difficult enough to trace without worrying about healthy carriers or nonparalytic patients. Even Wickman admitted that paralysis was still "the only sign which is characteristic of the disease; and . . . which conclusively establishes the diagnosis."[11] Although scientists had shown that the disease was contagious, cases were difficult to link together, particularly as polio investigators studied mostly paralytic patients.[12] These problems in identifying and tracing polio cases would continue to haunt epidemiological research into the 1930s and 1940s until the development of effective serological techniques.

The importance of understanding epidemic polio was made more urgent by the growing numbers of epidemics. By the late 1910s, researchers could cite reports of more than fifty-two epidemics, across Europe, the United States, and Australia.[13] A new element was added to polio's epidemiological picture after the most serious epidemic hit New York City in 1907, with an estimated 2,500 cases and a mortality rate of around 5 percent. New York neurologist Bernard Sachs headed an investigative committee that published its report on the etiology, pathology, and epidemiology of the epidemic in 1910. The section on epidemiology—written by a health official, a pediatrician, and a neurologist—reinforced many of Wickman's observations. They found that "general symptoms" could be as common as paralysis and that the disease spread along routes of travel. The extent of infectivity remained confusing: families usually had only one case, and cases were relatively evenly spread throughout the city. Because there were few adult victims, the authors concluded that polio was a "mild type of infection," strong enough to hurt children but not adults. Of 750 cases studied intensively they discovered only two black children, a "remarkable" and inexplicable finding.[14] The 1907 epidemic and the committee's report helped establish polio's new image as a disease associated with urban communities.

In large cities tracing direct contagion was even more difficult than in rural settings. Hidden, nonparalytic cases continued to confuse investigators and skewed case fatality rates so that an alarming proportion of the cases identified were reported fatal. Asymptomatic cases also made clinical diagnosis more difficult; now physicians and parents worried that every fever could be a danger sign, as they tried to distinguish the early symptoms of polio from other infant complaints.

American epidemiologists, however, continued to be influenced by Wickman's focus on small, rural outbreaks. One official, for example, urged epidemiological attention to rural epidemics for he believed that "epidemiologic evidence would be clearer cut in smaller places than amongst the complications necessarily encountered in a big city."[15]

Although American epidemiologists remained committed to the ideas and techniques of scientific medicine, their epidemiological work suggests that they were uncomfortable with some of its reductionist implications. In principle, the germ theory implied that contagion is random; but, in practice, researchers assumed a close relationship among disease, poverty, and filth. Their experience of epidemic polio did not significantly alter their traditional assumptions about the relation between disease and environment. In explaining the predictable and the anomalous, epidemiologists linked poverty and filth with the spread of disease, even when their evidence suggested that polio did not fit this pattern.

As William Coleman has shown in his recent study of yellow fever in the nineteenth century, examining the categories medical fieldworkers used to study disease enables us to piece together not only their assumptions about the nature of disease but also their concepts of the proper workings of a healthy society.[16] Polio researchers were faced with much puzzling evidence: Why was it so difficult to trace the connection between cases? Why were native-born, clean, and rich families affected as well as the immigrant, poor, and the dirty? Perhaps researchers could have begun to define this disease as *unlike* most other contagious diseases and unrelated to the filth of streets, homes, and persons. But they did not. When researchers found that poverty and filth did not seem to predict the appearance of epidemic polio, they did not suggest that good sanitation and living conditions were better predictors. Instead, they reinterpreted the appearance of cases in clean, suburban homes as random and sought to explain their spread by additional factors such as infected milk, insect vectors, and individual sanitary carelessness. Despite contradictory evidence, in epidemiological study as in public health work, polio remained firmly linked to filth and poverty.

MODELS IN POLIO EPIDEMIOLOGY

The models used by polio investigators reflected their experience with other endemic and epidemic diseases. Environmental factors, part of the nineteenth-century epidemiological repertoire, continued to be emphasized in the study of epidemic polio. Reflecting the long-standing link between public health

work and sanitary reform, polio researchers studied overcrowding, poor housing and living conditions, and other signs of
poverty and filth. They believed that poor immigrant families,
particularly those newly arrived from eastern and southern Europe, were likely victims and carriers. This focus on urban
slums partly countered Wickman's rural picture and reempha-
sized the danger of American cities. Like other Progressive reform movements it reflected not only an implicit nativism but
also the hope that with proper regulation the American city
could be made a pleasant and healthful place to live.

A second model was that of insect vectors. The successes of
medical entomology excited researchers who admitted that bacteriology had undermined the premise of environmental sanitation and sought pragmatic methods to integrate the germ
theory into public health work. Insects, visible to both physician
and parent, offered a way to explain the specific mechanism of
disease transmission and continued the link between public
health work, sanitary reform, and the filth theory. Yet this entomological model was also part of an emphasis by proponents of
the New Public Health on the responsibility of the individual; a
dirty child surrounded by flies was clearly a sign of parental
ignorance and carelessness.[17] Futhermore, disease-carrying insects with wings could also explain the presumed random appearance of cases. Especially apt for the spread of polio, this
model allowed officials to explain the appearance of paralytic
cases in middle-class homes otherwise assumed sanitary and
safe.

The third model emphasized direct contagion. It drew on the
scientific work of Flexner and other scientists who argued that
polio was spread by respiratory secretions. Since the germ
theory, health officials had expressed growing faith in controlling disease through identifying infectious agents and individuals. The case of Typhoid Mary, an Irish immigrant woman
found to be spreading typhoid fever as a healthy carrier in New
York City, had powerfully reinforced the connections between
ethnicity, class, ignorance, and germs. Polio epidemiologists recognized the importance of identifying and tracing individual
cases (a method known as shoe-leather epidemiology), but, with

no precise diagnostic test for polio, they found it difficult to establish evidence of direct contact between paralytic cases and those without clear symptoms. Wickman had undertaken detailed clinical epidemiology in small Scandinavian towns, but most American investigators faced polio epidemics in large urban communities where shoe-leather epidemiology was almost impossible. The selection of field groups thus became critical, and the choices investigators made reflected their assumptions that poverty and filth would explain the spread of this disease. Despite the integration of the new science of bacteriology into polio epidemiology, then, the long-standing fear of the poor and immigrants as sources of dirt and disease lingered.

TENEMENTS AND IMMIGRANTS

Nineteenth-century health reformers and sanitarians had associated the appearance and spread of disease with poverty and city life. American public health reformers Stephen Smith and Lemuel Shattuck used their work to critique the living and working conditions of the urban poor.[18] A focus on urban poverty seemed especially appropriate as epidemic polio began to appear in the major northeastern cities in the early 1900s. But American physicians and health officials found many inconsistencies in their attempts to classify polio as an environmental disease.

Most epidemiologists expected to find the majority of families with polio living in an environment filled with dirt, animals, and vermin. They assumed that their housing would be old, poorly built, with inadequate sewerage, probably large tenements or multifamily dwellings. But epidemiological work showed instead that many affected families lived in recently built houses, single family dwellings, or small tenement buildings and featured comparatively good domestic hygiene.

Researchers who studied urban outbreaks in the 1910s did find a link with the rural picture of earlier polio outbreaks. They found a higher incidence of epidemic polio in low density neighborhoods than in the tenements of Manhattan's Lower

East Side or the slums of South Philadelphia. In 1916, Manhattan and Brooklyn, highly congested areas of New York, experienced relatively less incidence of the disease than did the more sparsely populated boroughs of Queens and Richmond. Polio epidemics in cities like New York and Philadelphia offered a distinctly different picture from the rural farming communities Wickman had described. But researchers, nonetheless, began to identify rural characteristics of the disease, even within the great metropolis, New York.

In 1911 federal epidemiologist Wade Frost had pointed out that children from rural communities who developed paralysis tended to be older than those from urban neighborhoods. This crucial insight led him to consider that polio was not solely a children's disease. Frost compared polio to "certain other infectious diseases, notably measles, [which] are largely limited to children, not because they are essentially children's diseases, but because the adult population has been more or less immunized."[19] But Frost's rural factor was not pursued by epidemiologists until the 1930s and 1940s, for it suggested that clean suburbs might be more dangerous than crowded and dirty tenements.

The assumptions American epidemiologists made in exploring connections between polio and cleanliness became clear in a study of Staten Island during the 1916 epidemic. Staten Island (the borough of Richmond) had intrigued observers because it had the highest proportional incidence of epidemic polio of the five boroughs of New York. Yet Staten Island was relatively uncongested; its population density was as low as 2 persons per acre, compared with Manhattan's infamous 170. In 1916 epidemiologists from the U.S. Public Health Service conducted a detailed study of 328 affected Staten Island families. The researchers found their houses and surroundings clean, often with inside toilets, a sign of higher sanitary standards. Most of these families were native-born and lived "under suburban conditions." And, true to Frost's rural factor, they had the highest proportion of older children infected with paralytic polio. In fact, epidemiologist Allen Freeman believed, Richmond was "definitely separated, both geographically and in general character of life" from the rest of New York.[20]

In his additional study of polio cases in New Jersey and Connecticut, Freeman found that the economic standing of the families he investigated was not particularly low. He could discover "nothing significant" about the occupations of the householders, the phrase suggesting that this measure of class standing was also confusing. Even more frustrating for polio researchers was the limited evidence of direct contact, the result of the difficulty of identifying cases with mild symptoms. Federal officials found only one child in five had such a history.[21] Francis E. Fronczak, the health commissioner of Buffalo, similarly found only 18 percent of 273 cases during the 1916 epidemic "presented any history whatever of contact, even slight, directly or indirectly, with any previous case which could reasonably be taken as polio."[22] Epidemiologist Claude Lavinder concluded that the U.S. Public Health Service study of the New York City epidemic had not enabled him to determine polio's "precise mechanism of transmission and the avenues of infection."[23]

Lavinder and the other federal officers assigned to study the epidemic refused to consider the implications of their environmental investigations. Despite strong evidence of a correlation between suburban living, good sanitation, and the epidemic, Lavinder argued that the incidence of the disease was "relatively independent of local conditions" such as "density, economic status, and housing of the population." Polio, his colleague Wade Frost agreed, seemed to be distributed among "various elements" of the population unrelated to hygienic or economic conditions, race or nationality. "We are, in truth, quite ignorant as to the principles which underlie such phenomena," the U.S. Public Health Service researchers concluded.[24] Similarly, in a survey of twenty epidemics between 1907 and 1910, Joseph Collins argued that polio had nothing to do with unhygienic surroundings for "in some instances it was noted that the sanitary conditions were poor . . . but in the majority of epidemics such as those of Vermont, New York, Nebraska, Australia, and Westphalia, the hygienic conditions were good, and in some instances excellent."[25]

Although congestion and poverty did not seem to predict the appearance of epidemic polio, researchers nonetheless continued to expect that polio outbreaks would occur in over-crowded slum neighborhoods. This expectation also influenced their view of the ethnicity of likely victims and transmitters of the disease. The relationship between nativity and disease was a long-standing public health concern, heightened in these years of mass immigration. Although, in practice, polio epide-miologists found it almost impossible to identify carriers of the disease, their tendency to blame immigrants nonetheless sug-gests an underlying nativism. They expected the typical polio family to be poor southern or eastern European immigrants. But the affected families they found were often native-born or from established immigrant groups such as the Germans and the Irish. In the 1916 New York City epidemic around 30 per-cent of cases were native-born, 15 percent German and Irish, and 25 percent Italian and Russian. Worse, their children had higher mortality rates than those from Italian, Russian, or Pol-ish families. "Certainly," New York City's health commissioner reflected uneasily, "the social and economic conditions under which these people live are no more favorable than those un-der which the Americans, Germans and the Irish live."[26]

City and federal investigators tried to explain these perceived discrepancies by assuming that the ignorance of recent immi-grants skewed their results and made their answers unreliable. Allen Freeman, for example, believed that it was impossible to get accurate clinical histories because the "large foreign born population" with their "character and habits of life" made such evidence difficult to obtain and trust.[27] A New York City official found that of the 5,500 thousand cases he studied over 60 per-cent were from native-born families, and immigrant children with polio were well-cared for and previously strong and healthy. But he discounted this information as unreliable owing to the working-class origin of his informants; parents "of the poorer cases," he believed, "cannot give the same attention to detail as the well-to-do."[28]

Despite their evidence that a higher proportion of paralytic polio cases were children of native-born and middle-class fami-lies than immigrant families, investigators concluded that class and ethnicity played no part in determining the spread of the

Table 2. Nationality of Victims of Poliomyelitis Cases, 1916 Epidemic, New York City

	Manhattan	Bronx	Brooklyn	Queens	Richmond	Total in City
Native (born in U.S.A.)	822	386	1,873	583	161	3,825
Italian	402	58	684	161	41	1,348
Russian	494	79	685	25	4	1,287
Irish	231	47	277	76	13	644
Austrian	238	27	189	19	6	479
German	82	48	189	144	16	479
Polish	29	9	95	74	17	224
Norwegian	6	0	78	3	14	101
English	21	8	60	21	8	181
Hungarian	66	14	19	10	0	103
Rumanian	24	5	27	1	2	59
Scotch	12	1	27	6	0	46
Swedish	9	3	55	8	0	75
Lithuanian	1	0	13	0	0	14
West Indian	15	0	5	0	0	20
French	6	1	7	3	0	17
Danish	1	1	7	5	0	14
Canadian	10	1	5	3	1	20
Bohemian	12	1	0	5	0	18
Finnish	5	5	10	5	1	26
Syrian	1	1	6	1	0	9
Greek	14	0	3	0	0	17
Swiss	7	5	1	1	0	14
Spanish	8	0	4	0	0	12
Dutch	4	0	1	0	0	5
Turkish	8	0	2	0	0	10
Cuban	5	0	1	0	0	6
Japanese	1	0	1	0	0	2
Slavonian	1	0	1	0	0	2
Belgian	1	0	0	0	0	1
Puerto Rican	1	0	0	0	0	1
Portuguese	1	0	0	0	0	1
Mexican	1	0	0	0	0	1
African	1	0	0	0	0	1
South American	1	0	0	0	0	1
Indian	1	0	0	0	0	1
Armenian	2	0	0	0	0	2
Ukrainian	0	0	1	0	0	1
Total	2,540	700	4,326	1,154	285	9,005

Source: Haven Emerson, A Monograph on The Epidemic of Poliomyelitis (Infantile Paralysis) in New York City in 1916. Based on the Official Reports of the Bureau of the Department of Health (New York: Department of Health, 1917), 108–109.

disease. That is, they defined class as working-class, and ethnicity as only that of recent immigrants such as Slavs and Italians.
Their evidence, suggesting a link between the disease and other
nationalities, did not fit their preconceptions, and so it was
largely ignored. A traditional environmental model underlay
epidemiologists' questions but proved inadequate to explain the
patterns they found, for researchers were only willing to associate the disease with the presence—not absence—of poverty and
dirt.

THE APPEAL OF INSECTS

The new science of medical entomology seemed a promising way
to explain the spread of polio. The idea of insects as disease
carriers, a notion consistent with the New Public Health emphasis on domestic sanitation and individual responsibility, also had
a practical appeal. In 1913 Harvard public health authority Milton Rosenau argued that if the fly were the major culprit, then
the suppression of polio would be relatively easy, compared to
dealing with healthy carriers and missed cases where "the difficulties of the problem will be multiplied manifold." The health
officer, Rosenau reflected, "would prefer to know the precise
mode or modes of transmission of any disease rather than its
cause, or pathologic anatomy, or even its treatment." The evidence that polio cases rarely appeared in crowded institutions
like jails and orphanages convinced Rosenau that polio, unlike
an infectious respiratory disease, was probably spread by an insect, perhaps a fly or a bedbug.[29]

Polio epidemics generally appeared in late summer and
early fall and diminished with the beginning of winter. Initially
its seasonal appearance had raised the idea of infected dust.
Numerous researchers tried to correlate outbreaks with the
dry, dusty summer weather during which they often occurred.
After acknowledging that "we have gone into everything we
could think of" in investigating a 1908 outbreak in Minnesota,
Herbert Winslow Hill concluded that the dry weather and the
incidence of paralyzed colts suggested that dust infected with

horse manure could have spread the disease.[30] In a study of epidemics from 1907 to 1909 Massachusetts state officials also noted that polio epidemics often occurred during an unusually low rainfall. But, finding it difficult to measure quantities of dust, they pointed out that outbreaks also appeared in states with widely varying climatic histories and conditions.[31] Furthermore, a dust theory seemed uncomfortably close to the filth theory of disease. In his introduction to the U.S. Public Health Service report on the 1916 epidemic, Wade Hampton Frost acknowledged some experimental evidence showing that dust from a polio sick room had infected laboratory animals. But, he stressed, "to attach great importance to this mode of infection, however, would be foreign to our experience with other pathogenic microorganisms."[32]

Polio's seasonal characteristics also supported the theory that polio was spread by insects, perhaps flies that breed and travel more rapidly in hot weather. Inspired by the path-breaking work of Ronald Ross and Walter Reed, researchers hoped that medical entomology would be able simultaneously to answer puzzling questions about polio's spread and involve the latest laboratory research methods. In 1909 Hill warned that the "notorious errors made in the epidemiology of malaria and yellow fever in the days before [the mosquito] . . . serve as warning to make no final or conclusive statement regarding the epidemiology of polio."[33] In a U.S. Public Health Service report on polio, *What is Known of Its Cause and Modes of Transmission,* published during the 1916 epidemic, Frost acknowledged that polio's irregular geographic distribution, as well as its seasonal appearance, suggested that insects might play a part in its spread. That the majority of cases could not be "traced to known contact, either direct or indirect, with any previous case" had, he pointed out, led many investigators "to seriously doubt or even deny the transmissibility of the disease."[34]

In August 1916 the New York City Health Department hired an entomologist to study the city's polio epidemic. Charles Brues, an assistant professor of entomology at Harvard's Bussey Institute, began his search for an "intermediate agent" to help explain several "peculiar factors" about the epidemic. He drew on analogies with yellow fever and bubonic plague that had been shown to involve an insect or animal vector. The plague, which had appeared in California a decade before, particularly interested him, for it seemed to display epidemiological factors strikingly similar to epidemic polio: little relation to the density of population, and a tendency for cases to appear near waterfronts and on the lower floors of apartment buildings.[35] The rat flea had been suggested by another researcher who hoped it would resolve polio's epidemiological inconsistencies, for, added one man, "whoever has seen a city slum street in summer-time cannot imagine more intimate personal contact than is enjoyed by the tenement children playing in the crowded, hot, dusty thoroughfare, and yet it appeared that cases of infantile paralysis might be numerous in the tenements on one side of a street, with no cases whatever in similar houses opposite."[36] Brues, however, found it difficult to obtain conclusive evidence of rats and rat holes. He faced the legacy of previous polio investigations during which officials had reported households with unsanitary conditions to city agencies for prosecution. Many families, Brues found, had an "evident desire to deny the presence of anything not considered proper, or anything for which repressive measures might be required by the Department of Health."[37]

Brues considered the possibility of bedbugs, cat-fleas, sandflies, and houseflies, but he was most convinced by the laboratory research on stable flies. He cited his own experimental work and its confirmation by federal researchers at the Hygienic Laboratory in Washington. Brues warned that this research had not been fully confirmed and so was "not free from possible error."[38] Still, he felt that an insect vector was the most promising way to explain an epidemic that had "involved a population living under entirely different conditions from those existing in places where previous epidemiological investigations have been made."[39]

An insect theory helped to explain the appearance of polio among middle-class and nonimmigrant children. Insects, potentially, could spread disease randomly; it was not the fault of middle-class parents with a paralyzed child if an infected fly had traveled from the worst parts of the city. The disease, thus, could continue to be linked to dirt and the slums. Some-times these assumptions about class were made explicit. In 1914 two physicians argued, in support of their theory of blood-sucking insects as carriers of polio, that "observation demonstrates that constant distribution of the bedbug among members of various social classes takes place." They found examples of cross-class infection in a doctor attending a slum case, a lawyer in court, and a maid who spent her half-day off work in a tenement. The daily newspaper, they reminded readers, was distributed by tenement dwellers, and suburban families' laundry was washed by tenement laundresses. In such ways, they feared, it was possible to observe the "invasion of the American home."[40]

Even as Brues was concluding his study, however, the popularity of the insect theory of polio had begun to decline. In the September 1916 issue of the *New York State Journal of Medicine* Massachusetts health official Philip Sheppard told his medical audience that he did not believe that stable fly bites were "the only method of conveyance of this infection"; it was time "to enlarge upon the equally important possibility of personal contact."[41] In his 1916 report Frost also argued that, although the "traveling habits of the stable fly might appear to account for the occurrence of cases of poliomyelitis in persons at a considerable distance from the original source of infection," cases were not grouped together in places where flies were abundant, and diseases known to be insect borne were not "characteristically more prevalent in children than in adults, nor is there any obvious reason why they should be."[42]

Nonetheless, some physicians still used the entomological model to reinforce the link between class, germs, and dirt. A Kansas physician, visiting New York City during the 1916 epidemic, argued that doctors should trust the evidence of their own eyes, particularly when they found afflicted families surrounded by filth and insects. For, he urged, if "New York will screen its windows and doors you will possibly stop polio. . . . And in spite of the fact that we have been told and I suppose it has been accepted as true that insects and flies have nothing to do with the disease, still . . . if you will go on the Third Avenue

[E]L and go down town to the Battery you will see I don't know how many million windows and doors without screens."[43]

The entomological model appealed to many scientists, health officials, and clinicians. Laboratory research on disease-carrying insects was considered at least as precise as virological study of the polio virus. Scientists at Harvard Medical School, the federal Hygienic Laboratory, and at various city and state public health laboratories tried to identify polio vectors by testing flies and other insects. Although their results proved inconclusive, public health officials drew on this work to support fervent swat-the-fly campaigns during polio epidemics. And clinicians, denied a specific diagnostic technique like those for syphilis or typhoid, could search for insect bites on their patients and ask specific questions of parents and other household members about the extent of insect life. The entomological model allowed epidemiologists to trace the direct contact of cases, but at the same time it explained the so-called random appearance of cases in clean, middle-class families. Insects provided one way to integrate the environmental assumptions of reasearchers into the confusing picture of this disease.

DIRT AND DOMESTIC HYGIENE

In 1908 a Massachusetts health official argued that the discovery of polio's etiologic agent would clarify the way the disease spread. "Until the organism causing the disease is known," he commented, "it will be impossible to say whether the infection is carried directly to the patient or by means of food."[44] But his hope that etiologic identification would clarify epidemiology was, in the short term, ill-founded. Flexner's laboratory work suggested that the virus was transmitted by personal contact through sneezing or kissing. Some polio investigators welcomed this emphasis on direct contagion, for it associated the spread of the disease with personal hygiene. This association was both practical as well as intuitive; clean and careful families could protect themselves from disease. If the germs of polio were spread through unsanitary habits, then epidemiologists and health officials could explain epidemic polio in a way that was both convincing to the lay public and scientifically precise. In any case, urging individuals to control their domestic hygiene and personal behavior was part of a familiar public health litany, one not easily discarded. Nevertheless, as we have seen, investigators found it difficult to link the appearance of paralytic polio with a lack of cleanliness.

While a focus on germs may have in theory provided researchers with greater objectivity than a broad environmental model, investigators did not assume that the germs of polio spread randomly, irrespective of ethnicity or class. At a conference on polio during 1916, Haven Emerson reported the case of a doctor's child who had died of polio. He argued, however, that it was not an example of a physician bringing infection into his own family, for the child's Polish nurse was "the more probable carrier."[45] Similarly, Yale public health authority C.-E. A. Winslow explained the appearance of polio in an isolated wealthy family in Connecticut by the revelation that the family's chauffeur had been secretly visiting his sister in Brooklyn, a center of polio cases.[46]

Even more striking than the appearance of cases in the best families were the limited numbers reported among children living in charitable public institutions. During the 1916 epidemic in New York City, Haven Emerson found only ten polio cases reported from around 100 institutions with 21,000 children.[47] Only one researcher dared to suggest that this was owing to improved hygiene conditions in the institutions, where, he claimed, "cleanliness and discipline are carefully observed."[48] Most other observers fell back on isolation as the explanation by suggesting that only institutionalized children were thoroughly protected from the outside world. Still, in New York these institutions were forced to undergo massive sanitary campaigns, including the distribution of white muslin handkerchiefs for all children and increased bathing.[49] And although a study of polio patients from fifty-eight New York infant health stations found almost all were healthy, well-nourished consumers of pasteurized milk, this evidence of cleanliness did not dampen fears of dirt and contagion. No afflicted baby during the 1916 epidemic was permitted to attend an infant health station. New York health officials warned mothers about the importance of domestic hygiene; and no one from "infected premises" was allowed to "mingle unduly with the regular clientele" of any station.[50]

The case of Barren Island in New York's Jamaica Bay was another example of the shaky connection between polio and filth. At a number of discussions on polio, Haven Emerson pointed to this case to show that there was "no obvious or necessary causal relation" between environmental factors and the spread of the disease. Barren Island had 1,700 adults and more than 300 children, but the community reported no cases of polio. Yet the island was a sanitarian's nightmare: it had only shallow wells, and no sewage disposal or garbage collection was provided; the city sent the island most of its garbage and dead animals; and most of its population were Polish, Italian, and black unskilled laborers. It had, Emerson commented, "the most unpromising and insanitary conditions to be found within the limits of the city."[51] That polio had not appeared here was "remarkable," for "it is a place where one might expect the maximum of fly-carriage infection and maximum contact with serious garbage conditions."[52]

Another disturbing note was the consistently reported statistic of declining rates of infant mortality. After the 1916 epidemic Charles Bolduan, the director of New York City's Health Education Bureau, pointed out that infant mortality rates in the city were the lowest ever. It was the result, he believed, of effective public health education, which had helped officials gain public support so that the people obeyed health authorities. "The children have never before been so carefully watched over by their parents; never before have the parents been so mindful of the proper care of food and drink; never before have homes been kept so clean."[53] Other officials similarly believed that these figures were the result of their sanitary efforts, but they were amazed when this work did not protect families from polio. A New Jersey official noted that, at first, the 1916 epidemic appeared predictably among Italian, Polish, and Jewish families. But cases also occurred in a ward that his officers had taken "special pains" to clean three months previously; that ward had the greatest incidence of polio cases and the most deaths.[54] In 1917 Emerson commented privately to Flexner with a mixture of pride and bewilderment that, despite the previous year's polio epidemic with more than 2,400 deaths, the city's death rate as a whole had fallen four hundredths of a point below the crude death rate for 1915, with declining deaths from tuberculosis, typhoid fever, whooping cough, scarlet fever, measles, and infant diarrhea.[55]

Unwilling to link the appearance of the disease with healthy children and good sanitation, investigators sought external factors to explain the appearance of polio cases in families assumed sanitary and safe. The disease, they argued, must have entered middle-class homes from the outside. As polio was considered a child's illness, researchers urged particular attention to milk as a probable source of infection. Infected milk and water were, after all, familiar epidemiological subjects; they had provided health officials with the means to control cholera and typhoid. Parents were questioned closely about where children had obtained their food and drink; some feared immigrant peddlers were selling infected food to unwary middle-class children. A number of health officials adopted the infected milk theory. In New Jersey, for example, the Newark Health Department placed its milk supply under close surveillance throughout the 1916 epidemic.[56]

The strict quarantine and sanitation measures extolled by health officials as part of their anti-polio campaigns were seen by some observers to cross the line from the germ theory to the filth theory. These campaigns appeared jarringly old-fashioned, harking back to the days of sanitary science. Johns Hopkins researcher John S. Fulton complained that Maryland's statewide quarantine during the 1916 epidemic had shown that the public believed in "the spectacle of disaster" and that officials had reinforced "widespread misinformation and very embarassing fear."[57] Similarly, a New Hampshire physician criticized "backward" city health departments, whose efforts, he believed, were guided not by calm scientific leadership but fearful physicians and members of the public in "bondage to the superstition and discarded theories of a prescientific age."[58] "To judge from the almost hysterical quarantine measures instituted by various localities—in staid old Connecticut of all places," commented the editor of *Medical Record,* "one would think it as contagious as smallpox among the unvaccinated, or as yellow fever two decades ago."[59]

Proponents of the New Public Health had argued both that the lay public needed education to understand diseases were spread by germs, not filth, and that attention to personal hygiene, not quarantine, would protect against disease. A singularly contagionist view was voiced by a New York health official whose study of the New York City 1916 epidemic was funded by the Rockefeller Foundation. Alvah Doty, a proponent of the New Public Health, believed in the overriding danger of personal secretions in the transmission of disease for, he argued, "the true media of infection are discharged from the body containing infectious organisms in their active state."[60]

Doty stridently attacked other theories he found less scientific. "Nothing," he warned, "has contributed more to the extension of infectious diseases than erroneous theories concerning media of infection for they have encouraged carelessness in detecting the real means by which these maladies are transmitted from one person to another." He considered the standard polio epidemiological repertoire and rejected it completely: dust, horses, poultry, stable flies, rat fleas.[61] Unfortunately, Doty's attempt to prove that polio was spread by personal contact succeeded in only 10 percent of the 5,000 New York cases he studied. He justified this discrepancy, as Wickman had, by noting the difficulty of diagnosing the disease, particularly asymptomatic and mild cases; after all, "until recently this disease has not been well understood or clearly defined."[62]

Doty believed that hygienic carelessness and ignorance allowed infection into the home, and he specifically mentioned infected milk. But he found no evidence of infected milk in New York's general supply. To explain the fact that a large number of families with paralyzed children had used clean pasteurized milk he blamed irresponsible housewives. "The contamination of milk after it reaches the household is real and not imaginary," Doty warned, for it "easily become[s] a source of infection through want of proper attention to cleanliness." Immigrant and poor families, through "ignorance, overcrowding, bad sanitary conditions, and need of strict economy in the necessities of life" had brought disease upon themselves.[63] For, he wrote, that "among the poorer classes the person who prepares the food is often the one who tends the sick baby. . . . [Her] hands are more or less constantly contaminated with discharges, particularly from the intestinal tract, and there is no reason to believe that any special effort is made to ensure proper cleanliness. Therefore, even milk, although pasteurized, may become contaminated after reaching the home."[64]

Doty believed that the lay community, especially immigrants and the poor, did not fully understand the dangers of germs and the way they spread disease from person to person. He was disturbed to find that many members of the public still believed in the filth and miasmatic theories of disease. Like Chapin he agreed that one of the most effective weapons against disease was popular education. Perhaps polio could be conquered this way. "Outbreaks of infectious diseases," he argued, "cannot be successfully dealt with without the cooperation of the public and this cannot be gained unless the people have definite and reliable knowledge regarding the means by which these affections are transmitted."[65]

Physicians as well as members of the public were skeptical of such advice. Many agreed with William G. McAdoo, secretary of the treasury and public health, who commented in August 1916, that "this mysterious disease" had so far proven itself "beyond the control of science."[66] If polio could not be controlled, then perhaps its germ had not been definitively confirmed. Newark official Frederick Hoffman argued that "infantile paralysis is, broadly speaking, a new disease and the etiological factors are apparently exceedingly obscure."[67] Even public health authority William H. Park admitted that laboratories had not been useful during the 1916 epidemic, except for the diagnostic examination of spinal fluids. After all, he reminded a medical audience, "it can hardly be said that the germ has been identified," for there was still doubt about the virus identified by Flexner and Noguchi.[68]

Furthermore, not all physicians trusted the epidemiological evidence of limited contagion. In August 1916 physicians at New York's College of Physicians and Surgeons reported that scientists had "incomplete knowledge" of the disease and urged health officials to use measures "known to be effective in checking the spread of other infections."[69] In 1914, when Robert Lovett had a friend whose son was coming to Boston for polio treatment and wanted to stay with him, he wrote to Flexner to ask his advice. Flexner reassured Lovett about his concern for his eighteen-year-old daughter; "in such a case as you describe we should not withhold the person from returning to school or mingling in ordinary society. . . . On the other hand, I thoroughly understand your feeling and do not regard it as foolish, believing that I should have the same misgivings." Lovett replied that he had written "a perfectly frank letter to my friend . . . telling him that I supposed I was foolish, but that I did have a feeling that I would rather not have his boy at my house."[70] Similarly, Stanley Cobb, a Johns Hopkins physiologist, who spent the summer of 1916 in Cambridge with his wife and newborn son, later reflected that he had not been convinced about Flexner's viral theory, so "as a precaution against young Sidney's contracting the disease from bacterial contaminant, all four legs of the baby's crib rested in pots filled with water." The baby's room also was off limits to all but his parents.[71] Hospital staffs were cautious as well. In late July 1916, the father of five-year-old Paul Hughes of Staten Island drove his sick son to the Smith Infirmary in New Brighton. The boy died on the way, but the infirmary doctors at the hospital's morgue would not accept the body for fear that the disease would spread from the morgue to hospital patients. As it was too early in the morning for a health department to be open, for hours Hughes drove around Staten Island looking for someone to receive his son's body; finally an undertaker was granted permission to accept it from the Manhattan health department.[72]

A few investigators returned to the sign commonly noted by clinicians: intestinal symptoms appeared before paralysis. Federal official Allen Freeman suggested that an underlying reservoir of infection would probably explain the appearance of

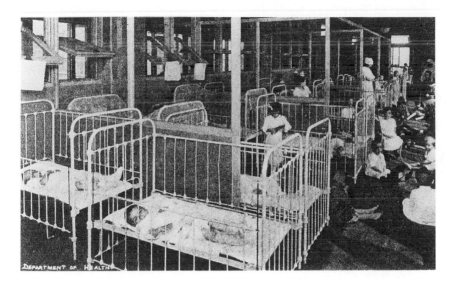

Fig. 11 Hospital staffs saw polio as contagious enough to warrant glass partitions (Haven Emerson, *A Monograph on The Epidemic of Poliomyelitis [Infantile Paralysis] in New York City in 1916. Based on the Official Reports of the Bureaus of the Department of Health* [New York: Department of Health, 1917])

polio epidemics, either animal or intestinal; the disease reminded him of contact typhoid.[73] C.-E. A. Winslow was not convinced by the idea of an insect host and proposed an intestinal factor; perhaps the germ of polio entered the body under lowered vital resistance, or perhaps infected food helped to spread the disease.[74] Wade Frost remarked that polio's seasonal appearance was the reverse of most respiratory ills that occurred in winter; polio, he thought, was more like a digestive tract infection.[75] However, these insights were largely overlooked, for they did not fit Flexner's conception of the disease, and the viral respiratory model was promoted by one of the most prestigious scientific authorities in the country.

Researchers were, not surprisingly, unwilling to believe that cleanliness itself might explain polio's epidemiological picture. Investigating poor sanitation was both familiar and practical, providing health officials with specific ways to educate the public. Doty's faith that a concerned housekeeper could guard her family from infection ignored previous epidemiological evidence that polio had attacked families with healthy, well-nourished children. In his study of outbreaks in New Jersey and Connecticut, Freeman found that sanitary conditions "were certainly as good as the average and perhaps better, and this is the most striking thing shown." Yet he argued that there was nothing to suggest that "the spread of the disease bears any special relation to the sanitary conditions under which it occurred."[76] The discrepancy between dirt and disease was the most difficult break from the traditional epidemiological past. Researchers explained the appearance of polio in middle-class homes by special factors such as careless parents who had allowed dangerous germs to enter their homes. The bacteriological model allowed investigators to transform dirt into infected filth, a sign that individuals, through carelessness and ignorance, had abdicated their responsibility for preventing disease.

But, despite the many conferences and theories, epidemiological research left health officials frustrated and unhappy. A North Carolina official complained that after the public adopted measures recommended by officials "they look to that officer for results." "I, for one," he continued, "do not believe that the present method of handling the epidemic is worth anything, hardly." The public blamed health officers when these measures failed to halt the disease, "and that is what they have a right to do, if we keep on with the present methods."[77] We should admit to travelers and people at home, an Alabama state health officer told his colleagues at a national conference on polio, that polio is a disease the medical profession knows "practically nothing" about and "that we are groping in the dark and are doing all we can to ascertain what is its cause and how it is disseminated."[78] Despite numerous epidemiological studies, physicians, health officials, and laboratory scientists were unable to explain the spread of the disease to their own satisfaction. "I do not think," Allen Freeman concluded at the end of another polio conference, "there is any disease which leads so much to a humble and contrite frame of mind as does poliomyelitis."[79]

This study of polio epidemiology between 1900 and 1920 suggests that the integration of the new sciences in epidemiological practice was shaped by traditional assumptions about the relationships among the disease, the environment, and the individual. Professional and popular acceptance of the germ theory coexisted uneasily with older ideas about the nature and cause of disease. In fact, the work of American epidemiologists reflected their belief that for epidemic polio the promise of the germ theory had not been fulfilled. The new tools of bacteriology had helped neither to clarify nor to control the disease, and no simple blood test or other precise way could distinguish infant summer complaints from the early or mild symptoms of this disease.

Despite Ivar Wickman's emphasis on the importance of asymptomatic cases, paralysis remained polio's determining symptom. Epidemiologists who traced mainly paralytic cases found their maps confusing, for they did not suggest a straightforward pattern of direct contagion. Drawing on their knowledge of other epidemic diseases, researchers tried to explain this confusing epidemiological picture by investigating housing and living conditions, class and ethnicity. But, unwilling to reject their environmentalist assumptions, epidemiologists chose to ignore correlations that did not seem to make sense. When they found polio cases among native-born, middle-class homes, they did not associate the disease with cleanliness or wealth. They expected polio cases to appear in working-class families who were recent immigrants, living in overcrowded, filthy conditions. The cases scattered among other members of the community were seen as anomalous.

To explain this random spread, researchers sought additional special factors that might have helped to carry infection to otherwise safe households. Their explanations, drawing on the New Public Health, stressed the importance of individual responsibility in preventing the spread of disease. Health officials' tendency to focus on the behavior of poor and immigrant families intensified their warnings about the danger of poor hygiene. Doty and other researchers blamed the "random" appearance of polio cases in middle-class families on house-keepers who had allowed tainted food, milk, or insects into their homes. Clearly, middle-class families were threatened by a dangerous outside environment as the daily interaction and services of immigrant families brought dirt and infection inside otherwise protected homes.

But in this case appealing to neither germs nor dirt helped to explain the spread of epidemic polio convincingly. Most major polio studies consistently challenged the traditional theories that held that overcrowding and poor sanitation spread disease. But, just as consistently, researchers concluded that hygiene, ethnicity, and class—as they defined these factors—had little or no relationship to the spread of epidemic polio. In one way they were right: the pattern of polio contradicted their given picture of epidemic disease. And no one chose to turn that picture upside down.

Epilogue: Polio Since FDR

During the 1920s and 1930s the public and the scientific community developed a new image of polio. Until then polio, seen as a children's illness that rarely attacked adults, was associated with immigrants and urban slums. Parents and physicians feared paralysis, polio's defining symptom, and scientists argued that it was primarily a neurological condition. The growing frequency and severity of polio epidemics and the difficulty of linking one case to another was explained partly by varying viral virulence, partly by children's vulnerability through trauma or focal infections, and partly by poor domestic hygiene.

This picture of the disease was gradually undermined. Polio came to be seen as a disease of cleanliness, occurring only among children who had been protected in early infancy from polio infection. Working with new strains of the polio virus, virologists began to argue that polio was not primarily a disease of the central nervous system but a systemic infection centered in the intestines. After epidemiologists discovered high levels of the virus in the sewage systems of Manhattan, New Haven, and other cities, they suggested that their evidence indicated widespread hidden infection. Polio's appearance in epidemic form, once every two or three years, was due to the infection of previously unexposed groups and the existence of more than one type of polio virus. Clean, protected middle-class children, they found, tended to have lower immunity levels of polio antibodies than poor children; this suggested that good sanitation provided dangerous barriers to natural infection.

These insights, derived from new techniques in virology and epidemiology, were also influenced by the appearance of a new cultural symbol, Franklin Delano Roosevelt, and reinforced by the work of the National Foundation for Infantile Paralysis, a national nonprofit organization headed by Roosevelt's former law partner, Basil O'Connor. Roosevelt's struggles helped recast the image of the cripple and removed much of the stigma from polio. The Foundation's massive efforts altered the direction of polio research by funding a new generation of virologists. Spurred by the Foundation's interest in applied research, American scientists developed polio vaccines, which, by the late 1960s, had reduced the number of paralytic polio cases and effectively ended polio epidemics in most American communities.

Yet, as our recent experience with AIDS suggests, diseases are not conquered so simply or easily. The story of polio raises important issues in disease history: the struggles among scientists and laymen to define and direct medical research; the role of popular heroes in reinterpreting the image of a disease; the ways popular expectations pressured physicians and philanthropists; and shifting concepts of the infected and disabled.

MAKING POLIO RESPECTABLE: THE ROOSEVELT YEARS, 1921–1945

The experience of one of America's most famous polio sufferers, Franklin Delano Roosevelt, did much to transform the public perception of the disease. No longer solely associated with poor immigrants, polio had struck a wealthy young man and created a cripple who nonetheless rose to the presidency. Furthermore, as a result of Roosevelt's experiences, the public began to perceive water as both cause and cure of the disease. In the 1930s and 1940s the National Foundation for Infantile Paralysis helped to solidify the newly respectable image of the disease and turned polio's treatment and research into a mass-marketing enterprise in which scientists no longer played the determining role.

The exact source of Roosevelt's infection has not been established, but numerous writers have pointed to his exhaustion during the summer of 1921.[1] Roosevelt traveled to his family's summer home on Campobello Island off the coast of New Brunswick, Canada. After various physical adventures, including falling into the chilly Bay of Fundy and helping to put out a local brush fire, Roosevelt developed the early symptoms of the disease and found he was unable to move his legs.[2] William W. Keen, an elderly specialist from Philadelphia who was vacationing nearby, told the family that this paralysis was probably the result of a blood clot on the spine, advised heavy massage as therapy, and sent a $600 bill. Massaging Roosevelt's sensitive legs was not only painful but also later believed to have exacerbated the paralysis. Another physician advised Keen to do a lumbar puncture immediately for diagnostic and therapeutic reasons, but the puncture was not done for another four days.[3] Finally Robert W. Lovett, a polio orthopedic specialist from Boston, was contacted. He advised hot baths instead of massage and diagnosed polio, but he suggested it was probably a mild attack.[4]

Roosevelt's experience with polio became part of his legend, a tale retold many times. His family and friends tended to play down any disabling emotional impact; Eleanor Roosevelt said its main effect was to accentuate her husband's already great power of self-control.[5] But the impact of paralysis on Roosevelt has intrigued many observers. Some have argued that his suffering transformed him and brought out hitherto hidden compassionate qualities.[6] Historians later suggested that polio gave Roosevelt a new image in the popular eye: "There can be no doubt of it, those months of pain put Franklin Roosevelt into the human race, and the permanent crippling that resulted from his disease kept him there. One no longer envied Roosevelt his headstart on life."[7]

Although it is difficult to trace a direct connection, after the publicity of Roosevelt's illness the public began to demonstrate a new fear of the swimming pools and public baths, which communities often closed during summer months when they feared an epidemic. Roosevelt himself may have seen water as both an infecting and therapeutic means, for, as he later told a friend, "the water put me where I am and the water has to bring me back."[8]

Water promised not only danger but cure. Roosevelt's faith in water therapy was spurred by an account of a young engineer who had regained the ability to walk after swimming in a pool at a Georgia health resort. Hydrotherapy had a long-standing and respectable medical past, particularly among America's elite.[9] The waters at this resort, with their high level of mineral salts and warm temperature, had supposedly held magical significance for local Native Americans and attracted numerous patrons before the Civil War.[10] After the war this resort town, later known as Warm Springs, drew guests mostly seeking relaxation rather than therapy. After an Atlanta journalist reported Roosevelt's visit in 1924 to the resort and his enthusiasm about the improvement in his leg muscles, other paralyzed patients began to flock to Warm Springs. Roosevelt became interested in revitalizing the resort and in developing polio therapy. His support of Warm Springs showed a typical combination of politics and philanthropy. In 1926 Roosevelt bought the property and grounds for more than $200,000, around two-thirds of his personal fortune, and a year later established a philanthropic foundation, of which he encouraged his friends to become trustees.[11]

Roosevelt's experience at Warm Springs has been considered another turning point in his life, as he encountered the popular view of the disabled. Living as a cripple among cripples clearly helped him adjust to his disability; but, at the same time, he experienced rejection by regular guests at Warm Springs.[12] Observers stressed that his friendship with fellow patients and his disdain for the regular guests' discrimination had a democratizing and liberalizing effect on Roosevelt.[13] Still, Roosevelt quickly became at ease in the racially segregated Southern resort, and Eleanor, rather than her husband, urged the building of the first local black school. There was no pool for black patients, but

Roosevelt later helped the nearby Tuskegee Institute establish polio rehabilitation facilities.[14]

Despite the strong connection in the public mind between Roosevelt and polio, Roosevelt did not significantly alter the popular image of the disabled. He did not get elected to Albany or to the White House as a handicapped person. During the 1920s Roosevelt argued publicly and privately that he would walk again, and his advisors energetically denied the extent of his paralysis.[15] But at the same time as he tried to deny it, Roosevelt also adapted his handicap into a political bargaining chip. In 1928, to aid Governor Alfred Smith's presidential campaign, Roosevelt was asked to run as Democratic candidate for governor of New York. He initially declined, citing his health as the reason, and retreated to Warm Springs. After he acknowledged the financial pressure created by his purchase of the spa, Democratic party chairman John J. Raskob offered to put up $250,000 to support Warm Springs. Only then did Roosevelt agree to run. This forged the initial links between Warm Springs, polio philanthropy, and its support by Roosevelt's wealthy political patrons that dominated Roosevelt's political career.[16]

Roosevelt found polio to be both a political asset and a liability. His political enemies used his affliction to boost rumors that he was physically, mentally, and morally unfit and that he exploited other polio victims.[17] After he became president, Roosevelt successfully enlisted reporters in a conspiracy of silence; they agreed not to describe or photograph him in his wheelchair or his leg-braces. The cameras of reporters who dared to breach this tacit ban were accidentally dropped, or their film was ripped out.[18] Many Americans were not even aware that their president was confined to a wheelchair; some political cartoonists portrayed Roosevelt running or jumping.[19] In the minds of many Americans, Roosevelt, a man who had overcome significant physical hardship and suffering, became a powerful symbol inspiring ordinary citizens during the Depression years.[20] Roosevelt, a polio victim from an elite family, helped to loosen the earlier link between polio, dirt, and the immigrant poor.

THE NATIONAL FOUNDATION FOR INFANTILE PARALYSIS: CHARITY AND
RESEARCH ON A LARGE SCALE, 1934–1958

A growing number of polio epidemics raised public awareness
that polio rehabilitation was becoming a national problem. In
the early 1930s a public relations firm suggested that the New
York Infantile Paralysis Commission raise money for polio patients across the country by holding a series of dances on the
president's birthday. Participants were exhorted to "dance so
that others may walk." The first set of Birthday Balls in January 1934 raised $1 million; the second netted $1.25 million of
which more than half was returned to local communities.[21]
These campaigns established the themes of later polio fund-
raising. Although connected to the Democratic party and the
president, the fund-raising events had no formal link to government or scientific agencies; they were organized at both the
local and national levels like other New Deal agencies but
based on volunteer work. Most projects were directed by philanthropic entrepreneurs, not doctors or scientists; and they
were advanced by sophisticated advertising techniques, particularly oriented around children as both potential victims and
donors.

Amid Roosevelt's political troubles in 1935 and 1936, the
public's sense that polio philanthropy was linked closely to the
Democratic party began to hurt these fund-raising efforts. In
September 1937 Roosevelt announced the establishment of the
National Foundation for Infantile Paralysis, an organization distinct from his Warm Springs Foundation. In November, during
a Hollywood fund-raiser, Eddie Cantor, a radio and vaudeville
entertainer, suggested that radio stations ask listeners to send
money to the White House and call the campaign the March of
Dimes.[22] The Foundation's campaigns were stunning successes,
based on the premise that polio had the potential to attack any
child, despite class or ethnicity.[23]

The Foundation maintained a close relationship with Hollywood. It enlisted the support of movie stars like Helen Hayes,
whose daughter had died of polio.[24] The Foundation also professionalized its fund-raising and publicity techniques and pro-

duced tear-jerker films like *The Crippler,* which starred the young actress Nancy Davis as a Foundation volunteer. By 1945 the Foundation had grown from a $3 million organization to one that had raised more than $20 million.[25]

REDEFINING THE VIRUS, 1920–1945

In the early 1930s medical journalist, muckraker, and former Rockefeller bacteriologist Paul de Kruif asked Arthur Carpenter, manager of Warm Springs: "Why do you use all that dough to dip cripples in warm water? . . . That doesn't cure them any more than it cured you or the President. Why don't you ask the President to devote a part of that big dough to research or polio *prevention?*"[26] De Kruif became secretary to the President's Birthday Ball Commission's scientific advisory committee and then, after the Foundation was established, secretary of its scientific advisory board, with a major role in directing the Foundation's research funds.[27]

The rise and fall of de Kruif's efforts in the 1930s epitomized the early failings of the Foundation's program. Basil O'Connor, president of the Foundation, initially rejected the traditional conservative approach of scientist-run research agendas and encouraged de Kruif to fund applied research. Unusual "microbe-hunters" and healers had always appealed to de Kruif.[28] He "fought hard against the scientific skeptics" and urged the Foundation to support Maurice Brodie, a young researcher whose work was backed by the elderly public health statesman William H. Park. In 1935 Brodie received $65,000 to produce and test a killed-virus polio vaccine that Brodie claimed was safe and effective. But the trials were a "deplorable debacle," de Kruif admitted later, for some vaccinated children developed paralysis possibly as a result of the Brodie-Park vaccine. Public suspicion of a polio vaccine was strengthened further by similar problems with a live-virus vaccine developed and tested by Philadelphia researcher John Kolmer.[29] Although Kolmer was not funded by the Foundation, the reports of both trials hurt the Foundation's reputation and pressured O'Connor into accepting that the Foundation's research agenda should stress basic science rather than polio cures.[30] De Kruif later resigned from the Foundation after a fight with the advisory committee over the funding of an Alabama nutritionist.[31]

By intensifying the popular faith in science and fear of the disease, the Foundation encouraged members of the public to donate their money and time. Its campaign techniques were unashamedly sentimental, going beyond the efforts of the American Heart Association, the American Cancer Society, and the National Tuberculosis Association. The Foundation exploited the emotional pull of crippled children, and March of Dimes posters and donation cans routinely featured a child on crutches. "The spectacle of a brave but paralyzed little child, boldly attempting his first steps with steel braces attached to his legs was well-nigh irresistible," a historian later commented.[32] But as public awareness and fear of polio increased, the Foundation's publicity created its own problems when the conquest of the disease was recast as a kind of holy quest.[33] Many American scientists were uneasy about the Foundation's glib upbeat promises of children learning to walk and researchers finding a polio cure. Scientists were told that for the Foundation to succeed, "a certain amount of flamboyant publicity was absolutely necessary and they must go along with it."[34] They saw the Foundation as the "sudden appearance of a fairy godmother of quite mammoth proportions who thrived on publicity."[35] Their greatest unease was probably derived from the fact that the directors of the Foundation were not scientists but laymen. But no fairy godmother could have avoided getting caught up in the territorial and professional battles within the scientific community, particularly those between older bacteriologists and the new generation of virologists.

The Foundation contributed significantly to the development of the discipline of virology in the United States. In fact, for American scientists, investigating the nature of the polio virus came to characterize virological research. Potential grantees quickly learnt to phrase their proposals to link them to part of the Foundation's polio research agenda. Nonetheless, one researcher later claimed that it would be "more than naive" to maintain that the "brilliant discoveries" between 1938 and 1953 were the "direct result" of Foundation support.[36]

During the 1930s and 1940s the basic scientific tenets about the nature of polio were undermined. The older model of polio research, epitomized by Simon Flexner's work, suggested that the polio virus entered the body through the nose and mouth and traveled directly to the brain and spinal cord along nerve pathways. This model of the disease boded ill for the development of a polio vaccine, for it was acknowledged that any vaccine grown from nerve cells could also cause brain infections such as encephalitis.[37] But by the early 1950s most scientists had come to believe that the polio virus only occasionally attacked nerve tissues. As young virologists developed ways to grow the virus outside neural tissues, they raised new hopes for the possibility of a safe vaccine.

The introduction of sulfa drugs and other antibiotics made tissue culture work more promising, as researchers could work without fear of bacterial contamination.[38] The most significant tissue culture work was conducted by John Enders, Thomas Weller, and Frederick Robbins at a newly established infectious disease laboratory at the Children's Hospital in Boston. In 1948, with a Foundation grant, Enders began to use a strain of polio virus known as the Lansing strain, which Charles Armstrong of the U.S. Public Health Service had found in 1939 would replicate in the brains of wild cotton rats and in laboratory-bred white mice. The Lansing strain was popular among younger virologists, although Flexner and other Rockefeller scientists continued to use the mixed MV strain.[39] Enders's team discovered that they could cultivate it in nonneurological tissue. The discovery of the new properties of the polio virus, along with ways to assess the appearance of the virus in tissue culture rather than through laboratory animals, cleared the way for safe vaccine production and won the team the Nobel Prize in 1954.[40]

These techniques also helped to resolve some complexities of polio immunology. Researchers had long recognized that certain patients developed polio antibodies in their blood. Contrary to the scientific model of other infectious diseases, these antibodies had not been linked directly to the disease, mostly because

Flexner had stressed the bloodstream's minor role in transmitting the virus through the body. To explain the appearance of paralytic polio among only certain groups of the population, some researchers argued that perhaps there was a widespread "natural" immunity against polio. But it was difficult to test these theories by conducting large-scale studies when researchers had to rely on a limited number of expensive laboratory monkeys.

Medical experience during World War II increasingly undermined the "natural" theory, as numbers of adults began to develop paralytic polio. Polio cases appeared among American soldiers in the Middle East, yet, local physicians claimed, the disease was rare among native adults. Furthermore, at home the demographic pattern of the disease was shifting, and polio victims were becoming older. In 1940 at least two-thirds of reported victims were younger than nine; in 1947 two-thirds were older than nine.[41] Using new serological techniques based on Enders's work, epidemiologists at the Yale Poliomyelitis Unit conducted large-scale studies that established a basic fact: although immunity was widespread, it was not "natural" but the result of subclinical infection. John Paul's 1949 study of two isolated Eskimo groups along the north coast of Alaska was particularly convincing. Other than a brief epidemic in 1930, these Eskimo communities had little exposure to polio. Paul found that no Eskimo younger than twenty had any polio antibodies, but that most Eskimos older than twenty—even those with no clinical symptoms—showed signs of infection in their blood. This evidence suggested that polio antibodies were a defining sign of exposure to polio and that such exposure might provide lasting immunity.[42] Thus, the Yale researchers combined epidemiological and laboratory-based techniques to develop a new concept of the disease.

Other work suggested that not only could the polio virus be grown on nonneurological tissue but also polio was not primarily a nerve disease. This new work was based on both new tissue culture techniques and new laboratory animals—the cynomolgous monkey and the chimpanzee; unlike Flexner's Rhesus monkeys, the animals could develop polio by being fed the virus.[43] In the 1940s and 1950s Dorothy Horstmann, David

Bodian, and Howard Howe found the polio virus in the blood of monkeys in the early preparalytic stages. Based partly on clinical comments that polio patients often had gastrointestinal symptoms, their work suggested that the blood played a major role in spreading the virus through the body and that the intestines rather than the brain and spinal cord might be the seat of the disease.[44] Most devastatingly, their work showed that Flexner's emphasis on the neurotropic nature of the virus was the result of his dependence on the MV strain of virus that had been artificially altered during years of passage through laboratory monkeys until it no longer held the same properties as "fresher" strains from recent human patients.[45]

Additional evidence also suggested that polio resembled an intestinal infection more than a respiratory one. Flexner's theory of the nose as the portal of entry was undermined by the disappointing results of a new polio preventive: a nasal spray. The anti-polio spray—tested in Alabama, North Carolina, Illinois, and Ontario, Canada, during the mid-1930s—neither stopped the spread of the disease nor protected children from infection.[46]

Particularly after what many commentators have seen as the hype of the later vaccine trials, polio historians have dwelt on Enders's laboratory work rather than the Yale epidemiological studies and stressed the appropriateness of his Nobel Prize. Unlike Salk, Enders has been portrayed as the model scientist, an independently wealthy New Englander, classically trained, modest, and self-effacing. Enders, observed one writer, epitomized "the ideal scientific investigator." His work with tissue culture required calm and patience: "a man in a hurry could not have made the discovery." It was "typical of Enders but in complete contrast to the dynamic hustle of subsequent polio research."[47] Enders had given up a prestigious position at Harvard Medical School to work at the Boston Children's Hospital, and one observer later argued that his modesty was "that of the true scientist with vision, who will always go for those subjects in his chosen field of interest that have the best chance of succeeding."[48] At the same time his team's success has also been presented as serendipitous. Commentators, echoing assessments of discoveries by Louis Pasteur and Alexander Fleming, have stressed that Enders used the embryonic tissue cultures he had "left over" from work on mumps.[49]

This era also saw new approaches to therapy. In the 1930s the Foundation began funding Drinker respirators, iron lung machines, which were first used in 1929 to help paralyzed patients breathe.[50] In 1940 Elizabeth Kenny, a charismatic nurse, arrived in the United States from Australia armed with a new theory and practice for training paralyzed muscles and a letter of introduction to Basil O'Connor. Although initially hesitant, the Foundation began to provide funding to train Kenny therapists after the University of Minnesota publicized her impressive results. Kenny, rejecting the prevailing medical emphasis on splints and lack of movement for paralyzed patients, urged instead the use of hot packs and active training of muscles. The skepticism of the established medical profession about her conception of polio as a disease that affected muscles and skin but not nerves put the Foundation in a difficult position.[51] American physicians saw the power of public pressure when the Foundation nonetheless trained therapists and nurses in Kenny techniques. The Foundation, however, refused to help Kenny establish a research institute to provide grants based on her theories of polio. The Kenny Foundation, established in 1943, became the only private grant agency for polio research and therapy that opposed National Foundation policy during this period.[52]

DEVELOPING VACCINES, 1946–1960

After World War II the National Foundation initiated a second major research push. Led by its new director of research, Harry Weaver, the Foundation encouraged polio researchers to debate issues in polio virology in a series of polio conferences "engineered in such a way that the independent-minded scientists would not know they were being directed."[53] In the 1930s and 1940s the Foundation had funded research on broad topics including the role of nutrition for polio prevention and possible chemical cures.[54] But, as Weaver adopted the view of younger virologists, he became increasingly antagonistic to the theory of polio as a neurotropic virus and more hopeful about the possibility of a polio vaccine. Weaver encouraged the funding of work in virological pathology and immunology, but, with this focus, the Foundation became embroiled in major disagreements among virologists over immunological theory and practice. At issue were the relative safety and efficacy of a live-virus vaccine, based on classic immunological principles, as opposed to a killed-virus vaccine.[55] A classic confrontation pitted virologist Jonas Salk, who believed that a killed-virus vaccine could induce effective immunity, against Albert Sabin, John Enders, and others, who argued that only a live-virus vaccine could raise antibody levels high enough to produce lasting immunity.

By the 1940s polio scientists could no longer speak of one polio virus. Researchers at Johns Hopkins and Yale showed that, as Australian scientist Macfarlane Burnet had suggested in the mid-1930s, there was more than one type of polio virus.[56] In 1949 the Foundation established a typing committee that funded young researchers to do the tedious work of confirming there were only three types.[57]

Jonas Salk arrived at the University of Pittsburgh in 1947; he sought independence and distance from the anti-Semitism that had hindered him from pursuing his career in more prestigious New York laboratories.[58] The Foundation gave him a grant to conduct polio virus typing tests. Salk had gained his knowledge of virology through work with Thomas Francis, Jr., at New York University and the University of Michigan. In 1942 Francis had developed a killed-virus vaccine against influenza, which had been used among American armed forces. But Francis had worried that the vaccine did not produce sufficient antibodies to create lasting immunity, and only troops forced to take booster shots formed the appropriate population for this kind of preventive measure.[59]

Using Enders's new tissue-culture methods, Salk developed a killed-virus polio vaccine that he initially tested on himself, his family, and institutionalized mentally and physically handicapped children.[60] In 1953 Salk and the Foundation decided to organize national trials to test his vaccine. Their decision horrified the more conservative members of the scientific establishment including Albert Sabin, who challenged the viability of a killed-virus vaccine and impugned Salk and his methods.

The Salk vaccine trials suffered from numerous professional and political troubles. Disagreements over the kind of control groups, the resignation of Harry Weaver, the role of the National Institutes of Health, and the choice of an objective assessor of the trial results all clouded assessment of the vaccine. Paul de Kruif contributed to the general unease by advising newspaper personality Walter Winchell two weeks before the trials to tell the public about the problems pharmaceutical laboratories had encountered in developing mass production techniques of the vaccine. Parly as a result of this publicity, around eighteen thousand children dropped out, but the trials, which lasted from April to June 1954, finally included the mass vaccination of 1.8 million children aged between six and nine in forty-four states.[61]

Most citizens, accustomed to big government and big enterprise during World War II, enthusiastically embraced the trials. The public appetite for a polio preventative had already been whetted by the gamma globulin trials of 1951 and 1952. Trials held in Utah, Texas, and Iowa demonstrated that injections of concentrated blood serum containing polio antibodies could provide six weeks of immunity, enough for one summer's protection.[62] Public fear had also been growing with the increasing severity of polio epidemics: in 1946 there were thirty-five thousand cases, and in 1952 fifty-eight thousand.[63]

As Foundation officials waited for the trial assessment report, it became clear that the results would not be available in time for the vaccine to be licensed and produced for the following summer. O'Connor decided to promise the commercial laboratories who had already retooled for vaccine production $9 million (around thirty-three cents a dose) to encourage them to produce the vaccine, agreeing to buy back the vaccine if the results were negative. He argued that if the vaccine received a federal license the first children vaccinated should be those who received placebos during the 1954 trial.[64]

On April 12, 1955, Thomas Francis, Salk's former mentor, presented his report on the trials at an open meeting organized by the Foundation and flooded with reporters. The date, the tenth anniversary of Roosevelt's death, was, Foundation officials claimed, simply coincidental.[65] Francis tried to limit sensationalism but conceded that the vaccine had been largely effective: it had protected 60 to 70 percent for the Type I virus, 60 percent for spinal paralysis, and most encouragingly, over 90 percent for the most debilitating kind of polio, bulbar paralysis. In his speech, however, Salk claimed that his new methods of vaccine preparation had eliminated even these small problems and that further killed-virus vaccines would be 100 percent effective. Salk's comments angered Francis and other cautious scientists already wary of Salk's participation in the Foundation's trial publicity. That same day a group of leading American virologists met to discuss the problems and possibilities of the vaccine, including questions about the strains Salk had chosen. After only two hours they voted to approve the vaccine, and it was immediately licensed by federal officials. The trials, a later commentator claimed, transformed the Foundation from a fund-granting agency to an active implementer of health strategies.[66]

The National Foundation turned Jonas Salk into a kind of Horatio Alger scientific hero. He was, their publicity brochures stressed, an inspiring example of a poor immigrant's son who had made good. The son of a Jewish garment manufacturer, Salk had graduated from New York's City College and received a medical degree from the New York University's College of Medicine.[67] Among many of his scientist colleagues, however, Salk was perceived as a publicity seeker. The Foundation's overwhelming support of his killed-virus vaccine only exacerbated relations within the virological community. In October 1953 at a meeting of the Foundation's immunization committee, although Sabin and others presented their continuing work on live-virus vaccines, the committee was cursorily informed by Foundation officials that such work was no longer of great interest to the Foundation. This, commented John Paul, a participant, resulted in an "open and sore wound."[68]

Both Salk's and the Foundation's reputations were briefly tarnished by what became termed the Cutter incident. Within fifteen days of Francis's April 1954 report, the Foundation's worst fears seemed to be realized when cases of paralysis were reported among children who had received the vaccine. After federal officials from the Communicable Disease Center established that these cases were the result of vaccination from a batch prepared by Cutter Laboratories of Berkeley, California, Surgeon-General Leonard Scheele halted the vaccination program for a week. By mid-summer 1955 Scheele had established a new Polio Surveillance Unit and had tightened vaccine testing requirements. Altogether 204 cases, including eleven deaths, were linked to the Salk vaccine, and forty suits for damages were later settled in California courts.[69]

Virologists initiated an investigation to determine whether the disaster was the result of improper laboratory methods or whether something in Salk's procedures had led to the appearance of live virus in the vaccine. This issue today remains unresolved. During meetings in June 1955, scientific experts voted eight to three to continue the vaccination program, but later they agreed that Salk had to find a substitute for the strong Mahoney Type I strain he had used. A few virologists, including John Enders, also attacked the "margins of safety" theory that Salk used to explain his method of inactivating the viral virulence. After Scheele's final report Eisenhower's Secretary for Health, Education and Welfare Oveta Culp Hobby resigned, and a year later so did Scheele.[70]

The development of a live-virus vaccine did not proceed smoothly either. Virologists Herald Cox and Hilary Koprowski had developed a live-virus vaccine at the Lederle Laboratories of the American Cyanamid Company. In 1950 they tested the vaccine on a group of mentally handicapped children at a New York state institution, despite the disapproval of Foundation science advisor, virologist Thomas Rivers.[71] Although critics questioned the ethics of calling these children "volunteers" and pointed out the possibility that the attenuated virus had reverted to virulence in vaccinated children's stools, both men continued separately to test their vaccines in Northern Ireland

and the former Belgian Congo. However, their vaccines began
to lose popularity after vaccine-linked polio cases were reported
in Northern Ireland, and the organizers experienced difficult
relations with the World Health Organization in Africa.[72]

Albert Sabin played a major role in attacking the Salk vaccine.[73] Born in 1906, Sabin was, like Salk, the son of immigrants, and his parents had come to New Jersey from Eastern
Europe when Sabin was fifteen. Placing himself firmly in American medical tradition, Sabin later claimed that he was inspired
to study medicine after reading de Kruif's *Microbe Hunters*.[74]
After graduating from New York University's College of Medicine in 1931, he worked at the Rockefeller Institute. Sabin left a
few years later, dissatisfied with Flexner's theories of polio, and
moved to the University of Cincinnati, where he conducted
numerous studies reinforcing the new model of the polio virus
as primarily intestinal.[75] In the mid-1950s he developed a live-
virus polio vaccine that he tested initially on himself, his family,
and two hundred federal prisoners. But by then the Foundation was committed to supporting Salk's vaccine. Sabin found it
difficult to obtain sufficient support to test his live-virus vaccine
in America; he noted that, in any case, the Salk vaccine had
altered the antibody levels of American children making an
adequate assessment of an additional vaccine impossible. In
1957, in a move unusual in the Cold War years, he announced
that a trial would be conducted in the Soviet Union.[76]

By the late 1950s polio work was increasingly supported not
by the National Foundation but by the Kenny Foundation and
the World Health Organization. These two groups funded polio conferences in 1959 and 1960 at which Sabin announced
that his live-virus vaccine had been tested with success on over
4.5 million people in the USSR, Singapore, and Mexico, compared to the 400,000 Americans and Western Europeans who
had received the Salk vaccine.[77] Sabin received international
acclaim, but United States federal officials still hesitated to
license a live-virus vaccine. In 1960, the Lederle-Cox vaccine
lost further popular confidence when paralytic cases occurred
after trials in Dade County, Florida, and West Germany.[78]
There were also disturbing reports of increases of polio cases

in communities vaccinated with the Salk vaccine. Salk explained these cases as the result of the public's failure to take
the right number of vaccine injections, an argument that
seemed to reinforce the appeal of Sabin's easy-to-take syrup.[79]
In 1961 the surgeon-general licensed the Sabin vaccine (and
later the Lederle-Cox and Koprowski vaccines), but, unlike the
fervent public enthusiasm in April 1954, this time there were
few public demonstrations. "The people had grown weary of
polio heroes," a later commentator reflected.[80]

The Sabin vaccine also encountered production problems, although there was no single Cutter incident. In 1962 the first
reports of Sabin-vaccine-associated paralysis appeared in the
United States. The cases were not just among the vaccinated, but
among children and adults who had become infected through the
stools of vaccinated children as the attenuated virus had mutated
into a more virulent strain. Although detective novelist Alistair
MacLean exaggerated when he described the invention of a mutated polio virus in *The Satan Bug* (1962) as "the most terrible and
terrifying weapon mankind has ever known," health officials acknowledged that a live-virus vaccine did pose some risk.[81] By
1964 federal officials had constructed a new polio vaccine policy
based on the acceptance of some risk; they suggested that initially
only those under eighteen and later only infants and preschool
children receive a live-virus vaccine. This new approach involved
instituting a reeducation program of the public to reverse the
Foundation's effective campaign that had urged every American,
young and old, to be vaccinated with the Salk vaccine.[82]

TELLING THE POLIO STORY, 1950–1990

The polio story has been told many times and for many different reasons. Like all good stories, it has something for everyone.
In the 1950s and 1960s it was a shining example of well-placed
optimism, showing that the public could safely trust science and
scientists. In the 1970s writers, dwelling more on the dark side
of the story, reflected the growing popular criticism, spurred by
Ivan Illich and Susan Sontag, of medical professionals and tech-

nology. In the 1980s polio commentators emphasized the human side to the making of science, the political and professional maneuvering that led to both mistakes and successes.

The Cutter incident remains a touchstone for historians. Some have blamed it on the speed of Salk's work and the decision to license the vaccine. The haste was seen as the result of the glitz of the Foundation's campaigns, its use of nonmedical personnel to direct science, and the cowering of scientists unused to the media's bright lights. The Foundation, in these accounts, became a force for evil. In the 1950s and 1960s, Aaron Klein argued in *Trial by Fury* (1972), "scientific endeavor was frequently reduced to the level of merchandising and the alleged objectivity of scientists was severely strained in the intensity of competition."[83] Klein blamed both the Brodie fiasco and the Cutter incident on the popular and political pressure from the Foundation that "forced a relaxation" of the meticulous, controlled methods of laboratory scientists and resulted in repeated tragedy before success.[84] A number of commentators have attacked the Foundation's attempt to alter what they perceived as the typical and virtuous values of academic science: caution, care, and a disdain for publicity. The development of the polio vaccine "was one of the worst kept secrets of the early 1950s," Yale epidemiologist John Paul reflected in his *History of Poliomyelitis* (1971). In viewing the Cutter incident, Paul concluded, "the degree of haste eventually exhibited by the foundation seems hardly to have been justified."[85] The public, stirred by the Foundation's campaigns, also contributed to this pressure. "In the atmosphere of triumph which prevailed it is doubtful whether the committee could have viewed the results of the field trial dispassionately." Even President Eisenhower suggested that public pressure for the Salk vaccine had probably caused scientists to "short cut a little bit."[86]

In this vision of the American scientific world, the early twentieth century has become a golden age, in which scientists were left alone and the public had faith inspired by ignorance and awe. In *The Fight for Life* (1938) science journalist Paul de Kruif argued that, before World War I, "hopes and doubts raised by their experiments had not yet touched the people.

The searchers themselves—though some of them foresaw that one day too this was going to become a people's death fight— still worked comfortably in the ivory towers of their laboratories."[87] Jane Smith, similarly, suggested in her recent study of the Salk vaccine, *Patenting the Sun* (1990) that the efforts of the Foundation, coupled with changes wrought by World War II, transformed the American scientific community from a closed world shaped by academic peer values to a new generation, more conscious of the values of the corporate world. This new generation demanded recognition outside the small circle of academe but still depended on the support and approval of colleagues trained in an older mold.[88] Science journalist Richard Carter in *Breakthrough* (1966) urged his readers not to blame those scientists who disliked the Foundation's methods, for scientists, he wrote, are "living creatures" and therefore resist change. "When something arises to alter the circumstances, threatens their prosperity, security and survival, they react negatively," he explained.[89] Smith, agreeing that the Cutter incident might have been prevented by more testing and less haste in releasing the vaccine, nonetheless concluded that "there were no clear villains to blame."[90]

In *Fighting Infection* (1977), a history of scientific conquests of the twentieth century, physician-historian Harry F. Dowling argued that "the conquest of poliomyelitis had all the elements of an American success story," with a straightforward objective "so obviously beneficial to mankind as to resemble the quest for the holy grail." It was, he argued, a crusade that enlisted "all groups and classes" and produced a popular hero whom he compared to David, "the killer of the giant." Yet, Dowling also suggested, this "sweet" victory "left a slightly bitter taste in many mouths."

> The obvious scrambling of several participants to be the first to win the race and the intemperate attacks by some who took up the cudgels on behalf of one or another of the chief actors smacked of the arena rather than the scientific laboratory. Perhaps this is the American way to success; if so, one can only hope that we will eventually learn to concentrate more on conquering nature than on outshining each other.[91]

Smith similarly implied that the Foundation's publicity methods—its large-scale use of radio, newsreels, and television—may have been too modern for old-fashioned scientists. This publicity, she suggested, might explain the lack of support for Salk by the mainstream scientific community. According to Smith, many of his colleagues felt that Salk was never "one of us."[92]

In the 1950s, Americans were tired of looking for communists; they wanted heroes. To some extent, this has been true for scientists and historians of science in recent decades as well. Polio storytellers seeking heroes have found Jonas Salk the obvious choice for Polio Prince, reflecting the lingering glow of Foundation publicity. Salk has been presented as both a model scientific researcher and a physician whose child subjects adored him and rejoiced to be vaccine volunteers—"the very model of the dedicated scientist."[93] But Salk is an ambiguous hero. In 1954 Salk, portrayed in the media as a typical self-effacing scientist, announced that he would no more "patent the sun" than the polio vaccine. But in fact, as Foundation lawyers had carefully established, no part of his vaccine procedure was new and could be patented. The scientific community saw Salk as a man seeking glory and fame, and there was some quiet satisfaction when the 1954 Nobel Prize committee for medicine announced not Salk's name but those of his scientific predecessors. Later observers suggested that the press conferences were also the reason Salk was not elected to the National Academy of Sciences.[94]

Smith has been one of the few writers to examine Salk's career beyond the vaccine trials. Salk wanted to establish an ideal institute, a "utopian intellectual community" to be filled with both scientists and humanists. But the Salk Institute for Biological Studies, built in La Jolla, California, with Foundation money, proved a disappointment to Salk. It became primarily a scientific research center, far from Salk's original conception, and was staffed by researchers who dismissed Salk as a "mere technician." At its opening in 1960, controversial popular attitudes to science were dramatically exemplified by local public demonstrations with charges ranging from antivivisection to anti-Semitism.[95]

When polio writers have taken the story beyond the Salk

vaccine they have felt impelled to compare the efficacy of
killed- and live-virus vaccines. Viewed retrospectively, Sabin's
vaccine has been mostly judged the "winner," offering more
solid and lasting immunity. The vaccine can also control epidemics because it can be taken quickly in its oral form. The Salk
vaccine, by comparison, has proven difficult to distribute and
administer in remote areas, requiring four or more doses de-
pending on the participants' level of antibodies.[96] But the live-
virus vaccine holds a predictable risk of paralysis; since the
resolution of the Cutter incident, the Salk vaccine, by comparison, has resulted in few vaccine-associated cases. Commentators
and polio policy makers today remain divided in their assessment of risk versus efficacy, although Sweden, Finland, and the
Netherlands have successfully conquered epidemic polio by using only the Salk vaccine.[97]

Writing on polio has frequently involved analyses of the process of research and the relations between funding agents, the
lay public, academic scientists, and the federal government.
The Foundation, most have acknowledged, tried to develop a
new kind of relationship between scientists and fund-raisers,
one in which lay directors actively shaped research programs
and saw themselves as public educators. The Salk vaccine trials
have been seen as the epitome of all that was wrong with this
approach. "The [1954] field trial has been taken out of its
proper setting as a scientific experiment of extremely difficult
and great magnitude and emerged as a dramatic spectacle,"
Paul argued. It was, he believed "a prodigious triumph" but "a
temporary disaster" for the reputation of American scientists.
Foundation research director Harry Weaver was wrong to organize polio conferences, Paul stressed, for scientists (at least in
the initial stages of their work) do not want to pool ideas and
prefer no outside interference.[98] The Foundation, further, has
been blamed for encouraging the public to develop unreason-
able expectations of polio scientists.[99]

Still, the polio story has largely been portrayed as one of
progress and success: Paul concluded his *History* by admitting
that "in spite of my efforts to tell the intricacies of the story in a
different, even dispassionate manner, it has been impossible to

avoid ending on a note of triumph."[100] As a result, most polio
chroniclers have ignored unsuccessful research tangents, such
as nutritional and chemical cures and Kenny's and the medical
establishment's competing models of polio therapy. Even Paul's
History, which offers a fairly balanced overview of these topics,
was, the author acknowledged, written by a polio participant
who actively contributed to current concepts of the disease.
Because the story of polio has been framed primarily by research scientists rather than by practicing health professionals,
we lack a sense of how physicians, other health professionals,
and families dealt with the disease. Apart from Salk, other major polio figures have been largely unexplored. There are no
full biographies of Sabin or O'Connor, and even the National
Foundation lacks a serious history. Many works, however, describe Franklin Roosevelt's polio experiences and discuss the
vaccine story itself.

As the polio story has long been considered one of scientists
and science, the public, except when portrayed as "victims" or
as a force tragically altering scientists' professional values, has
not been present in most accounts. Until recently historians
have largely ignored the roles played by women in the fight
against polio, although Smith noted the lay women volunteers
and organizers who supported the work of the Foundation.[101]
Some writers, particularly Roosevelt historians, have reflected
on the impact of polio on family relations. Roosevelt's affliction,
some have argued, was the making of Eleanor. Her husband's
paralysis forced her to expand the typical role of a politician's
wife and compelled her to take an active part in state and then
national politics.[102]

The increasing awareness among Americans of the rights of
the disabled may offer us another new perspective. Roosevelt's
Warm Springs resort has been described as "a community of
the handicapped," a place run by polio patients themselves,
structured around their own needs and desires, which often
contrasted sharply with those of able-bodied contemporaries.[103] Although Roosevelt may not have presented himself as a
handicapped leader, he helped to change the ways both American society viewed the disabled and the disabled viewed them-

selves. Alfred Smith reflected this when he supported Roosevelt's gubernatorial campaign in 1928 by saying, "A governor does not have to be an acrobat. We do not elect him for his ability to do a double back flip or handspring."[104]

Finally, the history of polio is clearly part of the history of disease in America. My study has mostly emphasized the early years, when polio's image was linked to recent immigrants and the filth and degradation of urban society. The work of the National Foundation, polio scientists (particularly epidemiologists), and the experiences of Franklin Roosevelt transformed this image of polio. The disease was, instead, seen as the "wages of virtue," the ironic result of a campaign to diminish infant mortality, which all too effectively helped American parents protect their children from germs and dirt.[105] "Epidemics of polio may be one of the prices we pay for civilization's advance," Roland Berg, a Foundation publicist reflected in 1949.[106] Ironically, polio remains in a way linked to dirt. In 1972 Aaron Klein noted that polio was conquered by a return to eating "dirty food" (sugar containing the live polio virus).[107]

The 1950s and 1960s were the high-water marks in the polio story. Despite the Cutter incident, the Salk and Sabin vaccines reinforced popular faith in the powers of science. Today medical speakers still refer to the victory over polio as an example of the lifesaving potential of scientific medicine. The massive publicity over the Salk vaccine trials, however, raised tensions in the scientific community over the ways the media transformed a scientist into a hero. When Enders and his team, but not Jonas Salk, were honored with the Nobel Prize the scientific community saw the choice as a comment on both Salk's role in the vaccine trials and the Foundation's unabashed campaigning. The National Foundation remains an important health funding organization today, but, with the expansion of federal research funding and other private health agencies, it lost much of its former prestige and influence. In 1958 the directors of the Foundation reoriented the March of Dimes campaigns away from an exclusive focus on polio to other health problems including arthritis and birth defects.[108]

In the last decade polio has been rediscovered by both scientists and the public. The popular and medical press have begun to report the surprising appearance of muscle weaknesses among older polio victims, a condition termed post-polio syndrome.[109] And, with the AIDS epidemic, the nature and control of infectious diseases have again caught the public imagination. The American experience of AIDS has raised health policy issues with some striking similarities to those of the past. We have seen the rise of popular and official interest in AIDS prevention and treatment only with the shift in the meaning and experience of the disease, as AIDS is seen to threaten not only gay bars and drug-ridden slums but also the homes and schools of middle-class heterosexual Americans. The American public has again turned to the laboratory and to scientists for understanding and hope. Jonas Salk, now an established virological statesman, has spoken encouragingly of the similarities between the polio and AIDS viruses in the search for an AIDS vaccine.

The story of polio in the United States is important not just because of its resonances with the recent experience with AIDS. Polio had a significant influence on U.S. medicine and science. Research on polio played a critical part in the development of virology and the training of the first generation of American epidemiologists. Through anti-polio campaigns public health officials expanded the methods of the New Public Health by demonstrating its persuasive power if not its immediate efficacy. Most important, polio epidemics influenced several generations of American doctors who faced a potential epidemic every summer, a disease that science could not prevent and barely treat. Even today there are no specific drug therapies for the acute stages of the disease. And, despite the impressive achievements of preventive polio vaccines, the appearance of post-polio syndrome suggests that other aspects of the disease remain problematic.

Polio's history is filled with ironies: public health campaigns that blamed dirty immigrants and lauded the preventive power of sanitation; flies that supposedly spread the polio germ by flying in only one direction, from the slums to the suburbs; researchers who interpreted polio's complex etiology and epidemiology by ignoring evidence that led them to middle-class, clean neighborhoods because it was the reverse of what they expected. Yet the American city was the locus of epidemic polio not because it was the center of physical and moral disorder, but because more families had protected their children from dirt and disease. Although an earlier generation of health reformers had feared that the germ theory would foster a sense of moral randomness in explaining disease, in the early twentieth century germs did not undermine moral and social determinants of disease. Epidemics made visible old and new ideologies, as health officials cleaned streets, preached hygiene, and tested sera and vaccines. Concerned citizens walked the streets distributing leaflets and sanitary advice. But their path was not random; it lead directly to the slums where Eastern European immigrants lived and worked. Their leaflets warned of the dangers of dirt, dust, and flies; disease was firmly located in the tenements and slums of the inner city. Epidemic polio raised potentially troubling questions when it appeared in safe and orderly environments and when its victims were from well-to-do native-born families. These questions were not resolved by blaming immigrants and translating germs into dirt.

Concluding his study of the 1916 epidemic, Haven Emerson reflected that, in some respects, the epidemic had been unproductive from an epidemiological point of view. Nonetheless, he concluded, "this disastrous visitation may yet turn out to be a blessing in disguise, if it fixes indelibly in our minds one obvious and incontrovertible truth—that the control not only of poliomyelitis but of all preventable diseases, does not depend upon the mysterious power of any supernatural agency, but that the remedy lies largely within ourselves."[110] Whether that agency be dreams, domestic healing, or laboratory research, Emerson's words bring the early history of polio closer to contemporary lives. We may no longer share pre-Rooseveltian assumptions about the carriers and victims of epidemic polio, but this story should caution us to persist in questioning the assumptions that underlie our definitions of disease today.

Notes

CHAPTER 1. GARDEN OF GERMS

1. Manton M. Carrick, "Preparedness: Our Best Weapon," *Southern Woman's Magazine* (1917), 28.

2. C. H. Lavinder, A. W. Freeman, and W. H. Frost, "Epidemiologic Studies of Poliomyelitis in New York City and the North-Eastern United States During the Year 1916," *Public Health Bulletin* 91 (1918): 24. See also John R. Paul, *A History of Poliomyelitis* (New Haven: Yale University Press, 1971); Saul Benison, "The History of Polio Research in the United States: Appraisal and Lessons," in *The Twentieth Century Sciences: Studies in the Biography of Ideas*, ed. Gerald Holton (New York: W. W. Norton, 1972), 308–343. By 1920 polio was officially reportable in Sweden, Norway, England, and the United States.

3. This is loosely drawn from Haven Emerson's description in "Transactions of a Special Conference of State and Territorial Health Officers with the United States Public Health Service, for the Consideration of the Prevention of the Spread of Poliomyelitis: Held at Washington, D.C., August 17 and 18, 1916," *Public Health Bulletin* 83 (1917): 26, hereafter cited "Transactions."

4. *New York Times*, July 6, 1916.

5. *Philadelphia Inquirer*, July 9, 1916; "Transactions," 13–48. Illinois, Ohio, and Massachusetts also reported cases into the hundreds. From July to September, Newark had 1,360 cases and 363 deaths; Charles V. Craster, "Poliomyelitis: Some Features in City Prevalence," *Journal of the American Medical Association [JAMA]* 68 (1917): 1535.

6. *Annual Report of the Department of Health of the City of New York for the Calendar Year 1916* (New York, 1917), Table 5, 117. In July the city had 777 deaths; in August, 1,078; in September, 364; and in October, 122. Previous

deaths from polio in New York City: 1912—70; 1913—54; 1914—34; 1915—13; *Annual Report*, 99. See also *New York Times*, July 5, 1916.

7. *Philadelphia Inquirer*, October 4, 1916.

8. See *New York Times*, July 14, 1916; *Philadelphia Inquirer*, August 15, 1916. In 1916 New York City had 108 black polio cases; Alvah H. Doty, *Special Investigation of Poliomyelitis 1916: Report of Committee Appointed by the Mayor to Cooperate with the Department of Health* (New York: Department of Health, 1916), 9–10; and see Haven Emerson to Simon Flexner, August 26, 1916, Polio file, Flexner papers, American Philosophical Society, Philadelphia; hereafter APS. Of cases in New York City, 30 percent were native-born; Doty, *Special Investigation*, 11.

9. Matthias Nicoll, Jr. "The Epidemic of Poliomyelitis in New York State in 1916," *New York State Journal of Medicine* 17 (1917): 270–274. Nicoll noted from 40 percent to 60 percent higher deaths among males than females.

10. Ibid.; and Nicoll, "Epidemiologic Data in the Poliomyelitis Epidemic in New York State," *Transactions of the American Pediatrics Society 29th Session* 29 (May 1917): 228–239.

11. In one cartoon a strong, healthy baby representing the Brooklyn Dodgers juggled seven puny men labeled as other baseball teams when the Dodgers were leading the National League, with the caption "No Infantile Paralysis Here," *Evening Bulletin*, August 23, 1916; in another, a notice·on a wall in front of the White House, in front of which boys symbolize the "Mexican Question" and a little girl the "Suffrage Issue," read "Quarantine against Paralysis of Business and Government" while an officer [Woodrow Wilson?] says, "Sorry! but I'm not taking any chances"; *New York Times Magazine*, August 13, 1916.

12. Andrew MacFarland, "The Treatment of General Infection by Sera and Vaccines," *New York State Journal of Medicine* 54 (1916): 229–232; Dr. Joseph Lebenstein, letter to editor, *New York Times*, July 18, 1916.

13. *Philadelphia Inquirer*, August 1, 1916. A Pennsylvania county medical inspector reported that during 1916 "the public has been kept in a state of constant unrest due to Prevention, Precaution and Preparedness"; *Eleventh Annual Report of the Commissioner of Health for the Commonwealth of Pennsylvania [for 1916]* (Harrisburg: J.L.L. Kuhn, 1920), 486.

14. See George Rosen, *Preventive Medicine in the United States, 1900–1975: Trends and Interpretations* (New York: Prodist, 1977), 16; Suellen M. Hoy, " 'Municipal Housekeeping': The Role of Women in Improving Urban Sanitation Practices, 1880–1917," in *Pollution and Reform in American Cities, 1870–1930*, ed. Martin V. Melosi (Austin: University of Texas Press, 1980), 173–198; and Phyllis A. Richmond, "The Germ Theory of Disease," in *Times, Places, and Persons: Aspects of the History of Epidemiology*, ed. Abraham M. Lilienthal (Baltimore: Johns Hopkins University Press, 1980), 84–93.

15. See, for example, Judith Walzer Leavitt, *The Healthiest City: Milwaukee and the Politics of Health Reform* (Princeton: Princeton University Press, 1982),

43–75; Martin V. Melosi, "Refuse Pollution and Municipal Reform: The Waste Problem in America, 1800–1917," in *Pollution and Reform in American Cities*, ed. Melosi, 110–120; James II. Cassedy, "The Flamboyant Colonel Waring: An Anticontagionist Holds the American Stage in the Age of Pasteur and Koch," *Bulletin of the History of Medicine* 36 (1962): 163–176; and Daniel Eli Burnstein, "Progressivism and Urban Crisis: The New York City Garbage Workers' Strike of 1907," *Journal of Urban History* 16 (1990): 386–423.

16. Paul Starr, *The Social Transformation of American Medicine* (New York: Basic Books, 1982), 135–136.

17. See George Rosen, *The Structure of American Medical Practice, 1875–1941*, ed. Charles E. Rosenberg, (Philadelphia: University of Pennsylvania Press, 1983), 41; and Starr, *Social Transformation*, 181.

18. See James H. Cassedy, *Charles V. Chapin and the Public Health Movement* (Cambridge: Harvard University Press, 1962); and George Rosen, *A History of Public Health* (New York: MD Publications, 1958); Starr, *Social Transformation*, 190–192. Charles V. Chapin outlined his major concepts of the New Public Health in *Sources and Modes of Infection* (New York: John Wiley & Sons, 1910); see also Chapin, *How to Avoid Infection* (Cambridge: Harvard University Press, 1917).

19. Cassedy, *Chapin*, 93–109.

20. On the still incomplete transformation of municipal public health work as a career in this period, see Charles E. Rosenberg, "Making It in Urban Medicine: A Career in the Age of Scientific Medicine," *Bulletin of the History of Medicine* 64 (1990): 163–186. See also Barbara Gutmann Rosenkrantz, "Cart Before Horse: Theory, Practice, and Professional Image in American Public Health, 1870–1920," *Journal of History of Medicine* 29 (1974): 55–73.

21. Hollis Godfrey, *The Health of the City* (Boston: Houghton Mifflin, 1910), 46. See Barbara Gutmann Rosenkrantz, *Public Health and the State: Changing Views in Massachusetts, 1842–1936* (Cambridge: Harvard University Press, 1972); and Russell C. Maulitz, " 'Physician versus Bacteriologist': The Ideology of Science in Clinical Medicine," in *The Therapeutic Revolution: Essays in the Social History of American Medicine*, ed. Morris J. Vogel and Charles E. Rosenberg (Philadelphia: University of Pennsylvania Press, 1979), 99–108.

22. For both New York State and City, see Anna M. Sexton, *A Chronicle of the Division of Laboratories & Research New York State Department of Health: The First Fifty Years, 1914–1964* (Lunenburg: Stinehour Press, 1967), 10–69; Arthur Bushel, *Chronology of New York City Department of Health (and its predecessor agencies) 1655–1966* ([New York: Department of Health]: 1966), 7–20; and John Duffy, *A History of Public Health in New York City, 1866–1966*, vol. 2 (New York: Russell Sage Foundation, 1974). See also Edward T. Morman, "Clinical Pathology in America, 1865–1915: Philadelphia as a Test Case," *Bulletin of the History of Medicine* 58 (1984): 198–214; Morman, "Scientific Medicine Comes to Philadelphia: Public Health Transformed, 1854–1899" (Ph.D. diss., Univer-

sity of Pennsylvania, 1986); and David A. Blancher, " 'Workshops of the Bacteriological Revolution': A History of the Laboratories of the New York City Department of Health, 1892–1912" (Ph.D. diss., City University of New York, 1979).

23. See Allan M. Brandt, *No Magic Bullet: A Social History of Venereal Disease in the United States Since 1880* (New York: Oxford University Press, 1985). On similiar problems for tuberculosis, see Rosen, *Preventive Medicine*, 11; and Barbara Gutmann Rosenkrantz, "Introductory Essay: Dubos and Tuberculosis, Master Teachers," in *The White Plague: Tuberculosis, Man and Society*, by René Dubos and Jean Dubos (New Brunswick: Rutgers University Press, 1987), xxiv–xxxi; and Georgiana Danielle Feldberg, " 'An Antitoxin of Self-Respect': North American Debates over Vaccination against Tuberculosis, 1890–1960" (Ph.D. diss., Harvard University, 1989).

24. In 1910, when the Rockefeller Institute's Hospital buildings were opened, cases of infectious disease were housed in a separate building with a complex crossventilation system, "the emphasis on removal of noxious air was actually a survival of antiquated notions about the conveyance of infections"; George W. Corner, *A History of the Rockefeller Institute, 1901–1953: Origins and Growth* (New York: Rockefeller Institute Press, 1964), 95. A designer for the Johns Hopkins Hospital in the 1890s similarly proposed a special building for infectious cases, suggesting that when the building became a dangerous source of pollution it could be pulled down; Charles E. Rosenberg, *The Care of Strangers: The Rise of America's Hospital System* (New York: Basic Books, 1987), 137–139.

25. See Elizabeth Fee, *Disease and Discovery: A History of the Johns Hopkins School of Public Health and Hygiene, 1916–1939* (Baltimore: Johns Hopkins University Press, 1987); John Ettling, *The Germ of Laziness: Rockefeller Philanthropy and Public Health in the New South* (Cambridge: Harvard University Press, 1981); and Elizabeth W. Etheridge, *The Butterfly Caste: A Social History of Pellagra in the South* (Westport: Greenwood Press, 1972).

26. "Transactions," 78.

27. For the appeal of flies in explaining polio, see Paul, *History*, 291–299. For the link between flies and immigrants, see Terra Ziporyn, *Disease in the Popular American Press: The Case of Diphtheria, Typhoid Fever, and Syphilis, 1870–1920* (Westport: Greenwood Press, 1988), 85–86; and Naomi Rogers, "Germs with Legs: Flies, Disease and the New Public Health," *Bulletin of the History of Medicine* 63 (1989): 599–617.

28. Susan Eyrich Lederer, "Hideyo Noguchi's Luetin Experiment and the Antivivisectionists," *Isis* 76 (1985): 31–48; Corner, *Rockefeller Institute*, 84–87. On Flexner's social and intellectual life, see James Thomas Flexner, *An American Saga: The Story of Helen Thomas and Simon Flexner* (Boston: Little, Brown, 1984).

29. Corner describes Flexner: "Reserved, seemingly impersonal, he was the embodiment of scientific efficiency; but behind the cool exterior there was an unsuspected breadth of mind and a sympathetic heart"; Corner, *Rockefeller Institute*, 36, also 154–158. For a less complimentary picture, see Saul Benison, *Tom Rivers: Reflections on a Life in Medicine and Science* (Cambridge: MIT Press, 1967), 122–132.

30. *New York Times*, July 9, 1916. For the need to demonstrate to John D. Rockefeller and the public that progress being made, see Corner, *Rockefeller Institute*, 158–159. On Noguchi, see Isabel R. Plesset, *Noguchi and His Patrons* (Rutherford: Farleigh Dickinson University Press, 1980).

31. Corner, *Rockefeller Institute*, 24–28. On the Phipps Institute for Tuberculosis in Philadelphia, the McCormick Institute for Infectious Diseases in Chicago (1903), and the Hooper Institute for Medical Research in San Francisco (1914), see Corner, *Rockefeller Institute*, 52, 150–151.

32. *New York Times*, June 2, 1901; cited in Corner, *Rockefeller Institute*, 38.

33. Corner, *Rockefeller Institute*, 43–46, 56–61. See also Ettling, *Germ of Laziness*, 181–184; and E. Richard Brown, *Rockefeller Medicine Men: Medicine and Capitalism in America* (Berkeley: University of California Press, 1979).

34. *New York Times*, March 12, 1911; cited in Paul, *History*, 116. On American antivivisectionists, see Lederer, "Noguchi"; and Corner, *Rockefeller Institute*, 87, 96–97, 159.

35. Corner, *Rockefeller Institute*, 111–114; Benison, *Rivers*, 116–119; and Sally Smith Hughes, *The Virus: A History of the Concept* (New York: Science History, 1977), 75–78. In the early years of virology, filterability was the only way to differentiate viruses from bacteria.

36. Benison, *Rivers*, 116, 144. Polio is a primate-specific disease. Only humans and monkeys share the gene containing a surface protein that enables the polio virus to bind and grow. It is one of the few viruses with such properties; herpes, for example, will grow in any animal.

37. Flexner and Noguchi, "Experiments on the Cultivation of the Virus of Poliomyelitis," *JAMA* 60 (1913): 362; Flexner and Paul Lewis, "Experimental Epidemic Poliomyelitis," *Archives of Pediatrics* 27 (1910): 95–96. On Noguchi's ability to discover ways of cultivating etiological agents that other scientists found extremely difficult if not impossible to reproduce, see Benison, *Rivers*, 144; and Corner, *Rockefeller Institute*, 113, 266. For this 1913 announcement Flexner was nominated for the Nobel Prize by William W. Keen; see Benison, "History of Polio Research," 315.

38. On some of these debates, see Paul, *History*, 156; and Benison, *Rivers*, 135–138.

39. Paul, *History*: "Flexner soon went off on several unrewarding tangents, pursuing his own theories," 431.

40. Saul Benison, "Poliomyelitis and the Rockefeller Institute: Social Effects and Institutional Response," *Journal of the History of Medicine* 29 (1974): 75.

41. Benison, *Rivers*, 193. "I don't know how many years were used up in debating whether the portal of entry was the nose or mouth. Progress was held up purely by chance because a big man like Flexner was using the rhesus monkey"; *Rivers*, 193.

42. Scientists today believe that there are three main types of the polio virus, but Flexner argued strongly that there was only one type, although the idea of types was already acknowledged by those who developed pneumonia vaccines. See Benison, *Rivers*, 192–193.

43. Paul, *History*, 156. See also Benison, *Rivers*, 145.

44. On the conflicts between Rivers and Flexner, see Corner *Rockefeller Institute*, 264–266. Rivers, a pediatrician turned virologist, joined the Institute in 1922 and later became director of its hospital.

45. Paul, *History*, 374–381; see also Paul F. Clark, "History of Poliomyelitis Up to the Present Time," in *Infantile Paralysis: A Symposium Delivered at Vanderbilt University April, 1941* (New York: National Foundation for Infantile Paralysis, 1941), 3–33.

46. Paul, *History*, 108, 117–119; on Flexner's inflexibility, see A. McGehee Harvey, *Science at the Bedside: Clinical Research in American Medicine, 1905–1945* (Baltimore: Johns Hopkins University Press, 1981), 93–95. Paul argued that Flexner's experimental path led him "deeper into the woods," *History*, 117.

47. Survey evidence from Charles-Edward Amory Winslow, "The Laboratory in the Service of the State," *American Journal of Public Health* 6 (1916): 222–233; and see Ira V. Hiscock and Margaret Scoville Hiscock, "Public-Health Laboratories," in "Report of the Committee on Municipal Health Department Practice of the American Public Health Association in Cooperation with the United States Public Health Service," *Public Health Bulletin* 136 (1923): 162–167.

48. *Newark Evening News*, July 6, 1916; and see "Medicine Wages Fight Against Unseen Infantile Paralysis Germ," *Philadelphia Inquirer*, September 10, 1916.

49. "Experience" [letter to editor], *Evening Bulletin*, August 10, 1916.

50. See Rosen, *A History of Public Health;* Rosenkrantz, "Cart Before Horse."

51. Paul, *History*, 149–151; Charles Bolduan, "Haven Emerson: The Public Health Statesman," *American Journal of Public Health* 40 (1950): 1–4.

52. See James G. Burrow, *Organized Medicine in the Progressive Era: The Move Toward Monopoly* (Baltimore: Johns Hopkins University Press, 1977);

Rosemary Stevens, *American Medicine and the Public Interest* (New Haven: Yale University Press, 1970); Starr, *Social Transformation.*

53. See Rosen, *Preventive Medicine;* Judith Walzer Leavitt, "Public Health and Preventive Medicine," in *The Education of American Physicians: Historical Essays,* ed. Ronald L. Numbers (Berkeley: University of California Press, 1980), 250–272. See also Fee, *Disease and Discovery;* and Greer Williams, "Schools of Public Health: Their Doing and Undoing," *Milbank Memorial Fund Quarterly* 54 (1976): 489–527.

54. [C.-E. A. Winslow], "Milton Joseph Rosenau," *American Journal of Public Health* 36 (1946): 530–531.

55. See Charles-Edward Amory Winslow, *The Life of Hermann M. Biggs: Physician and Statesman of the Public Health* (Philadelphia: Lea & Febiger, 1929). See also John R. Paul, *An Account of the American Epidemiological Society: A Retrospect of Some Fifty Years* (New Haven: Yale Journal of Biology and Medicine: Academic Press, 1973), 71; and Cassedy, *Chapin,* 97.

56. Abraham M. Lilienfeld, "Wade Hampton Frost: Contributions in Epidemiology and Public Health," *American Journal of Epidemiology* 117 (1983): 379–383; and Philip F. Sartwell, "The Contributions of Wade Hampton Frost," *American Journal of Epidemiology* 104 (1976): 386–391.

57. See Starr, *Social Transformation,* 134–135, 18.

58. For a somewhat different argument, see Nancy Tomes, "The Private Side of Public Health: Sanitary Science, Domestic Hygiene, and the Germ Theory, 1870–1900," *Bulletin of the History of Medicine* 64 (1990): 509–539. Tomes points to the blurred divisions between sanitary and bacteriological conceptions of disease. For nineteenth-century assumptions, see Charles E. Rosenberg, *The Cholera Years: The United States in 1832, 1849, and 1866* (Chicago: University of Chicago Press, 1962).

59. My thinking about dirt was first stirred by Mary Douglas, *Purity and Danger: An Analysis of the Concepts of Pollution and Taboo* (London: Routledge and Kegan Paul, 1966); but see also Cassedy, "Flamboyant Colonel Waring"; Lloyd G. Stevenson, "Science Down the Drain: On the Hostility of Certain Sanitarians to Animal Experimentation, Bacteriology, and Immunology," *Bulletin of the History of Medicine* 29 (1955): 1–26; and Charles E. Rosenberg, "Florence Nightingale on Contagion: The Hospital as Moral Universe," in *Healing and History: Essays for George Rosen,* ed. Rosenberg (New York: Science History Publications, 1979), 116–136. For the links between the modernization of dirt and middle-class American standards of virtue, see Starr, *Social Transformation,* 189, 192.

60. I found two instances for 1916: a New Jersey high school swimming pool was closed, *Newark Evening News,* July 19, 1916; and a physician warned against swimming in the Hudson River and East River, *New York Times,* July 5, 1916. Epidemiologist Paul argued that water does not play a significant role in the transmission of polio; see *History,* 283.

CHAPTER 2. THIS DREAD SPECTRE

1.   Ethel M. Barry, "The Bond of Motherhood," *New York Times*, August 17, 1916, verse 2 of 4.

2.   See Richard A. Meckel, *Save the Babies: American Public Health Reform and the Prevention of Infant Mortality, 1850–1929* (Baltimore: Johns Hopkins University Press, 1990), chaps. 1, 5. In 1916 New York City had around 9,000 polio cases, but there were more cases of chicken pox (9,600; around 9 percent of all cases reported); diphtheria (13,500; more than 10 percent); tuberculosis (19,000; more than 15 percent); syphilis (20,126; more than 15 percent); and measles (21,000; more than 15 percent); *Annual Report of the Department of Health of the City of New York for the Calendar Year 1916* (New York, 1917), 60, Table 1. The number of deaths from polio was high (2,448) exceeded only by those from tuberculosis (8,406).

3.   *Evening Bulletin*, July 5, 1916; see also *Newark Evening News*, July 5, 1916.

4.   The Charity Organization Society postponed fresh air outings indefinitely; *New York Times*, July 8, 1916. And see an advertisement by the New York Association for Improving the Conditions of the Poor, "10,000 Vacations Wanted," *New York Times*, July 12, 1916. The association also cited a quotation from Emerson: "One of the best things the New York Association . . . can do to co-operate in efforts to control the epidemic of infantile paralysis is to extend its fresh air work . . . for the children of the tenements"; *New York Times*, July 13, 1916.

5.   William Harvey Young to Blanche Debra Young, July 8, 1916 (letters in possession of James Harvey Young, Decatur, Georgia).

6.   Young to Young, July 21, 1916.

7.   Miss Martha Moore to E. Louise Sands, quoted in Sands's letter to editor, *New York Times*, July 28, 1916. In poor districts, streets were nearly deserted, and windows were filled with children being kept indoors by parents; *New York Times*, July 8, 1916.

8.   *New York Times*, August 10, August 13, 1916. See also letters to the editor, *New York Times*, August 13, 1916. After a death in a Staten Island neighborhood, a family with a young son "were planning to keep the little fellow away from all of the other children entirely. It seems to me that it is the only safe way to deal with such a treacherous matter. Were the children who come to us not in such close contact in the street, it would be well to close our school, I am sure. But as it is, I guess it is well to carry it on"; Young to Young, July 27, 1916.

9.   Samuel G. Dixon, "Summary of the Pennsylvania State Work in Poliomyelitis," *JAMA* 68 (1917): 90.

10.   *Evening Bulletin*, July 13, 1916; *Philadelphia Inquirer*, August 4, 1916. Dixon quarantined all children under sixteen entering the state from localities where the disease existed unless they brought health certificates. Special in-

spectors were empowered to search all points of entry, all railroad cars, vehicles, steamboats, and ferries. In both New Jersey and Pennsylvania health officials called on railroad companies to disinfect their cars regularly; *New York Times*, July 8, 1916.

11. *New York Times*, July 11, 1916. The "wealthy residents" of Islip, Long Island, posted a large red sign; *New York Times*, August 11, 1916.

12. *New York Times*, July 8, 1916; see also *Newark Evening News*, July 20, 1916.

13. *Newark Evening News*, July 14, 1916.

14. *New York Times*, July 20, 1916; "Transactions," 30.

15. *New York Times*, July 15, 1916; *Philadelphia Inquirer*, July 29, 1916. The federal certificate stated that a traveler with children under sixteen years of age had to present "a satisfactory health certificate from the health authorities at point of departure that his premises are free from poliomyelitis (infantile paralysis). The children accompanying traveler have been inspected and show no evidence of that disease." Copy of certificate, Record Group 90-1712, Box 157, National Archives, Washington, D.C.

16. Visiting nurses employed by the New York City Health Department, for example, were expected to send certificates to notify the health department and a sick child's school of any case of infectious disease and to hang placards inside and outside the patient's home; see *Rules for Employees of the Bureau of Preventable Diseases: Including Those for all Employees* (New York: Department of Health, 1915), Section 104, 59.

17. See *Evening Bulletin*, August 7, 1916. Parents flocked to Philadelphia's City Hall for certificates.

18. In July the U.S. Public Health Service (USPHS) warned those who dealt with polio patients to disinfect all clothing, bed linen, excretions, and the sick room itself; *Philadelphia Inquirer*, July 22, 1916.

19. An editor noted that there was no known length of infection; *New York Times*, July 6, 1916.

20. *Newark Evening News*, July 7, 1916. Dr. Ellwood Kinley, a Philadelphia physician, suggested enforcing an immediate embargo on all freight from New York unless properly disinfected and urged officials to take the same precautions as against yellow fever, where "even the mail is disinfected"; *Philadelphia Inquirer*, August 5, 1916.

21. *Evening Bulletin*, August 8, 1916; *Philadelphia Inquirer*, August 9, 1916. Dixon charged Camden officials with "promiscuously" issuing certificates; Camden officials denied the claim. Rail companies announced that they would require a health certificate from every traveler under sixteen before they would sell a ticket; *Evening Bulletin*, August 7, 1916.

22. Winifred Welles, "The Little Lepers," *New York Times*, August 6, 1916. This poem appeared on the editorial page.

23. *New York Times,* July 6, 1916.

24. *Newark Evening News,* July 5, 1916.

25. *Philadelphia Inquirer,* August 11, 1916.

26. Cornell University postponed its opening for two weeks; *Evening Bulletin,* August 31, 1916. Princeton University delayed opening from September 26 to October 10; *Philadelphia Inquirer,* August 19, 1916; and the U.S. Military Academy at West Point banned all children under sixteen from entering its grounds; *Philadelphia Inquirer,* July 9, 1916.

27. *New York Times,* July 6, 1916. Emerson sent a letter to every rector and pastor in the city and warned them not to admit children from infected homes to church gatherings. In Jersey City clergymen were told to close Sunday schools; *New York Times,* July 7, 1916.

28. Young to Young, July 14, 1916.

29. Quoted from *Newark Evening News,* July 19, 1916; see also *New York Times,* August 10, 1916.

30. *New York Times,* July 16, 1916.

31. Duffy, *Public Health in New York City,* 265. By the 1890s this image had begun to change as some private patients entered the hospital; Rosenberg, *The Care of Strangers,* chap. 10.

32. *New York Times,* July 5, 1916.

33. *Philadelphia Inquirer,* August 6, 1916.

34. *New York Times,* July 2, 1916; *New York Times,* July 8, 1916.

35. *Newark Evening News,* July 15, 1916. F. H., in a letter to editor, *Evening Bulletin,* August 22, 1916, protested that the "poor people of this city" have to "submit to outrage" of quarantine.

36. *New York Times,* July 26, 1916. The White Plains Common Council, for example, refused to have a private isolation hospital built and ordered all local children with polio—from both poor and wealthy families—to be sent to the public Westchester County Hospital; *New York Times,* August 12, 1916. See also Leavitt, *The Healthiest City;* and Rosenberg, *The Care of Strangers.*

37. In New York City, of 1,809 cases admitted to twenty-eight hospitals, 1.5 percent were falsely diagnosed as polio, and the mortality rate was 17.5 percent. Haven Emerson, *A Monograph on The Epidemic of Poliomyelitis (Infantile Paralysis) in New York City in 1916. Based on the Official Reports of the Bureaus of the Department of Health* (New York: Department of Health, 1917), 263; hereafter cited *Monograph.*

38. *New York Times,* July 8, 1916.

39. "The mothers are so afraid that most of them will not even let their children enter the streets, and some will not even have a window open," Martha Moore to E. Louise Sands, in Sands's letter to editor, *New York Times,* July 28, 1916. Louis C. Ager, a Brooklyn physician, warned that germs did not

travel through air and urged parents to keep windows open; *New York Times*, July 7, 1916.

40. Moore to Sands, *New York Times*, July 28, 1916.

41. *Newark Evening News*, editorial, July 12, 1916.

42. *Newark Evening News*, July 14, July 17, 1916.

43. *Newark Evening News*, July 18, July 8, 1916. Patterson officials also closed Sunday schools and barred Boy Scouts from their regular matinee at a Patterson movie show.

44. *Newark Evening News*, July 12, 1916; *Philadelphia Inquirer*, August 1, 1916. Krusen forbad a street dance that would be part of a local carnival; *Evening Bulletin*, August 30, 1916.

45. *Evening Bulletin*, August 19, 1916.

46. *New York Times*, August 11, 1916.

47. *New York Times*, August 10, 1916.

48. *New York Times*, August 10, August 11, 1916. In Philadelphia Krusen called off the annual baby show at Woodside Park; *Evening Bulletin*, August 7, 1916. Quote from *New York Times*, August 10, 1916.

49. *New York Times*, July 4, 1916. The ban was reported: "BAR ALL CHILDREN FROM THE MOVIES IN PARALYSIS WAR."

50. *New York Times*, July 4, 1916; *New York Times*, July 6, 1916; *Philadelphia Inquirer*, July 6, 1916. Krusen warned three movie houses that unless they agreed to exclude children under sixteen voluntarily they would be closed down; *Philadelphia Inquirer*, August 15, 1916. Emerson mentioned that Mayor Mitchel was resisting "tremendous pressure" from real estate agents and apartment house owners who wanted placards warning of the presence of cases removed; *New York Times*, August 11, 1916.

51. *Evening Bulletin*, July 8, 1916.

52. "Infantile Paralysis Prevented by Cleanliness" [advertisement]; *Evening Bulletin*, September 11, 1916: "Disease germs cannot live in its presence. Use it in water when scrubbing floors, windows and doors, and in disinfecting sick rooms, closets and drains. It also kills fleas, flies, bed bugs, roaches, ants, moths and all insect pests."

53. *Philadelphia Inquirer*, July 20, 1916. Less specific was the Mountain Valley Water Company's Radium Water, which could "protect the children and yourself" for it "eliminates waste and drives poisons from the blood, therefore protects against many diseases including INFANTILE PARALYSIS"; *Evening Bulletin*, August 23, 1916.

54. *New York Times*, August 4, 1916.

55. *Philadelphia Inquirer*, August 4, 1916.

56. *Evening Bulletin*, July 10, 1916. These activities involved the Health Department, the Street Cleaning Department, the Police Department, and the

Tenement House Commission. Ten million gallons of water were used nightly to flush streets and alleys in South Philadelphia; *Philadelphia Inquirer,* August 16, 1916.

57. The writer of a feature article in the *New York Times Magazine* reminded readers that the last major polio epidemic in the East, in 1907, had centered on New York and Boston, areas with a high concentration of immigrants from Northern and Eastern Europe; *New York Times Magazine,* July 9, 1916.

58. In response to a rumor that the New York epidemic had been imported from Italy, a story circulating in the city after cases were first reported among Brooklyn Italian immigrant families, Haven Emerson contacted the Harbor Quarantine Station and requested information about any cases of polio among incoming Italian immigrants. The Quarantine Station had not seen any signs of the disease, but Emerson continued to pursue the matter with federal officials in Washington; *Newark Evening News,* July 6, 1916. In Newark garbage was selectively removed in sections "inhabited by foreigners"; *Newark Evening News,* July 19, 1916.

59. Emerson, *Monograph,* 17; *New York Times,* July 1, 1916. The Department of Social Betterment of the Brooklyn Bureau of Charities issued one hundred thousand leaflets printed in Italian, Yiddish, and English; *New York Times,* July 9, 1916. The Rockaway Board of Health issued circulars in English, Italian, and Slavic; *Newark Evening News,* July 8, 1916.

60. *Philadelphia Inquirer,* July 9, 1916. Wilson signed the Siegal Resolution allowing Ellis Island facilities to be used as a hospital; *New York Times,* July 12, 1916. There were few explicit reports of anti-Semitism: ninety-eight Jews from New York were quarantined for three weeks at Wyckott's Mills, New Jersey; *Newark Evening News,* July 19, 1916.

61. *Evening Bulletin,* July 6, 1916; see also *Philadelphia Inquirer,* August 4, 1916: "While proper sanitary conditions, local authorities insist, are least favorable to the culture of the germ, yet, apparently they are not impassable barriers to its development."

62. *Eleventh Annual Report of the Commissioner of Health for the Commonwealth of Pennsylvania,* 488. A large number of cases in New York City and other cities had been in "immaculately kept apartments in clean neighborhoods"; *New York Times,* August 6, 1916.

63. Editorial, "Ambassador Page," *New York Times,* August 14, 1916. Her death showed forcibly the "utter darkness in which scientists are groping." There was also concern over cases appearing in the Upper East Side of New York, "which from its location and character was believed to be immune from an epidemic of this kind"; *Philadelphia Inquirer,* August 1, 1916.

64. *Evening Bulletin,* July 31, 1916.

65. See advertisement by local jewelers: "In their Efforts to Help Stamp Out Infantile Paralysis Will Furnish Free to Picnic Parties or Excursions Sanitary Drinking Cups FREE for the Asking"; *Newark Evening News,* July 12,

1916. On soda fountains, see *New York Times,* July 8, 1916; on disinfected sandboxes, see *New York Times,* July 8, 1916.

66. See a notice from the Charity Organization Society with suggestions to salesmen, expressmen, delivery men, and others obliged to enter districts where polio was prevalent: wear clothes that can be washed, wash face and hands, use antiseptic nose and throat douches, use antiseptic dentifrice as tooth powder, and shampoo hair at least once a week; *New York Times,* July 14, 1916.

67. See, for example, *Philadelphia Inquirer,* August 20, 1916.

68. *Philadelphia Inquirer,* August 1, 1916; *Evening Bulletin,* August 9, July 31, 1916; *New York Times,* July 12, 1916.

69. *Evening Bulletin,* August 22, August 18, 1916.

70. "Transactions," 81.

71. *Evening Bulletin,* July 14, 1916. See also Flexner, [abstract], "The Nature, Manner of Conveyance, and Means of Prevention of Infantile Paralysis," *New York Medical Journal* 54 (1916): 168–169. See also "Infantile Paralysis a Scourge and a Puzzle," *New York Times Magazine,* July 9, 1916, quoting Flexner on the dangers of coughing, kissing, sneezing, contaminated secretions from nose and mouth, uncooked food, and house flies.

72. See also instructions by William Rucker, assistant surgeon of the U.S. Public Health Service; *New York Times,* July 8, 1916. Rucker also noted the importance of dust and insects.

73. Editorial, *New York Times,* July 6, 1916.

74. "Bureau of Public Health Education," *Annual Report New York City 1916,* 83–85; *New York Times,* July 8, 1916. Films included "Long Haul vs. Short Haul" on the advantages of breast feeding; "The Price of Human Lives" on tuberculosis; and "The Life History of the Fly," 83.

75. *New York Times,* July 5, 1916. The mayor of Philadelphia said the police would help in Dixon's cleanup campaign by identifying those who had violated state and local laws about the disposal of household refuse, but that citizens shouldn't wait for the flying squadron of inspectors; *Philadelphia Inquirer,* August 5, 1916.

76. *Philadelphia Inquirer,* July 24, 1916.

77. *New York Times,* July 6, 1916.

78. *Newark Evening News,* July 6, 1916.

79. *Newark Evening News,* July 14, 1916.

80. "Guard the Babies," editorial, *Evening Bulletin,* August 3, 1916.

81. *Evening Bulletin,* July 22, 1916. After reports that the disease was "as prevalent among children in better families as among underfed and ill-kept children," Krusen said that this meant the campaign to control the epidemic would prove more difficult than "under other circumstances"; *Philadelphia Inquirer,* August 4, 1916.

82. *New York Times Magazine,* July 9, 1916.

83. *Evening Bulletin,* August 31, 1916.

84. *Philadelphia Inquirer,* July 23, 1916.

85. *New York Times,* August 12, 1916. The organizations that provided the nurses included the Association for Improving the Condition of the Poor, the Charity Organization Society, the Henry Street settlement, the United Hebrew Charities, and the United Jewish Aid.

86. Emerson, *Monograph,* 38, 40. Of more than ten thousand families visited, thirty-three nurses found only nine unreported cases of polio; for details, see 39.

87. Magistrates' fines ranged from two to five dollars; *New York Times,* July 11, 1916.

88. Moore to Sands, *New York Times,* July 28, 1916.

89. "Guard the Babies," *Evening Bulletin,* August 3, 1916.

90. *Philadelphia Inquirer,* August 5, 1916.

91. *Newark Evening News,* July 17, 1916.

92. Editorial, "A Revival of Shot-Gun Methods in Epidemic Control," *American Journal of Public Health* 6 (1916): 932–933. This piece mentioned officials' warnings about housecleaning, pets, vermin, flies, food, and personal contact.

93. Ibid. A Newark health official also admitted that many public health efforts were simply pragmatic, for those to whom the public looked for help had nothing to offer, but "on the other hand, if we wait for a load of monkeys to be imported for us to experiment on, our precautions may be taken too late"; *Newark Evening News,* July 22, 1916.

94. S. S. Graves, letter to editor, *Evening Bulletin,* September 14, 1916.

95. *Evening Bulletin,* July 6, 1916.

96. *Philadelphia Inquirer,* July 25, 1916.

97. *Evening Bulletin,* August 17, 1916.

98. *Handbook of the New York State Exhibit at the Exhibition of the Fifteenth International Congress on Hygiene and Demography at Washington, D.C., September 16–October 5, 1912* (n.p., n.d.), 86. See also the reference to "Exhibit of Culture of Pathogenic Bacteria Isolated from Vagrant House Flies," ibid.

99. W. H. Frost to Surgeon General, October 25, 1911, Research Group 90-1712, Box 157, National Archives. Frost also collected spinal fluid, material from two autopsies, several animals suffering from paralysis, and tonsil and adenoid growths from children who might be "healthy 'virus carriers.' " Dixon and other officials cited "conclusive" work from other state laboratories that showed the role of dust, which could carried from sick room to nursery; *Evening Bulletin,* July 22, August 17, August 30, 1916.

100. Young to Young, August 14, 1916.

101. Forty-four branches of the New York Public Library were closed to children under sixteen, and if a returned book was found to have come from an infected home, it was burned; *New York Times,* July 18, 1916. Newark public libraries were also closed; *New York Times,* July 9, 1916. On fomites, see a Newark health official: "Flies, bedding, clothing, anything that comes into contact with an infected person may become a carrying agent"; *Newark Evening News,* July 10, 1916. Notice by Charity Organization Society to delivery men: "See that door knobs, telephones and other frequently handled objects in your office are washed daily with a disinfectant"; *New York Times,* July 14, 1916.

102. Charles-Edward Amory Winslow commented that he could still see in his mind's eye the Dickens novel that was supposed to have given him measles as a child; Winslow, *The Conquest of Epidemic Disease: A Chapter in the History of Ideas* (1943; reprint, Madison: University of Wisconsin Press, 1980), 369.

103. *New York Times,* July 8, 1916; Emerson, *Monograph,* 45; *Philadelphia Inquirer,* August 9, 1916. Philadelphia's chief of housing reminded the public that science had already shown that domestic cats carried the germs of diphtheria and scarlet fever and might carry those of polio as well and so should be exterminated; *Philadelphia Inquirer,* August 7, 1916.

104. "Transactions," 33; *New York Times,* July 1, July 4, 1916. On the work of the Women's Society for the Prevention of Cruelty to Animals, see *Philadelphia Inquirer,* August 9, 1916.

105. *New York Times,* July 30, 1916. Dixon warned families to wash all domestic cats and dogs in a 2 percent solution of carbolic acid; *Philadelphia Inquirer,* July 19, 1916. See also Philip E. Sheppard, "Acute Epidemic Poliomyelitis: A Contact Infection," *New York State Journal of Medicine* 16 (1916): 445.

106. G. M. Bentley, "Benefits to be Derived from Observing, Collecting, and Studying Insects," *Tennessee State Board of Entomology* 20 (1917): 4.

107. *Newark Evening News,* July 16, 1916. The ad continued: "Make your home safe from the invasion of disease germs from the outside and from the breeding of disease germs within./ Do this the same way big hospitals do it. *Use Lysol*/ . . . Use it in toilets, wash bowls and everywhere flies and insects gather and breed."

108. For a more detailed explication of this idea, see Rogers, "Germs with Legs," 599–617. A belief in flies as disease carriers became so established a part of the New Public Health that satirical novelist Sinclair Lewis used the "Fly Week" as an example of the work of Almus Pickerbaugh, a scientifically irresponsible populist public health director; Sinclair Lewis, *Arrowsmith* (1925; reprint, New York: New American Library, 1961), 215, 248.

109. See Rogers, "Germs with Legs," 605–613; and L. O. Howard, *The House Fly: Disease Carrier: An Account of Its Dangerous Actions and of the Means of Destroying It,* 2d ed. (New York: Frederick A. Stockes, 1911).

110. See *Infantile Paralysis in Massachusetts, 1907–1912* (Boston: Wright & Potter, 1914). And see Charles J. Brues, "The Relation of the Stable Fly (Stomoxys Calcitrans) to the Transmission of Infantile Paralysis," *Journal of Economic Entomology* 6 (1913): 101–109.

111. Paul, *History,* 299–301.

112. See M. J. Rosenau, "The Mode of Transmission of Poliomyelitis," in *Infantile Paralysis in Massachusetts, 1907–1912* (Boston: Wright & Potter, 1914), 86–95.

113. See *Investigations on Epidemic Infantile Paralysis: Report from the State Medical Institute of Sweden to The XV International Congress on Hygiene and Demography, Washington 1912,* translated by Alfred V. Rosen (Stockholm: State Medical Institute, 1912).

114. Wade H. Frost, "Notes on the Discussion at the Fifteenth International Congress on Hygiene and Demography," *Public Health Reports* 27 (1912): 1661–1664. For less enthusiastic work, see W. A. Sawyer and W. B. Herms, "Attempts to Transmit Poliomyelitis by Means of the Stable-Fly (Stomoxys Calcitrans)," *JAMA* 61 (1913): 461–466. These California researchers doubted that the fly was the "usual agent in spreading the disease in nature." They suggested that screened sick rooms should be added to measures against contact infection but that they should "not [be] substituted for them," 466.

115. John F. Anderson and Wade H. Frost, "Transmission of Poliomyelitis by Means of the Stable Fly (Stomoxys Calcitrans)," *Public Health Reports* 27 (1912): 1733–1735. Compare their more critical study, Anderson and Frost, "Further Attempts to Transmit the Disease through the Agency of the Stable-Fly (Stomoxys Calcitrans)," *Public Health Reports* 28 (1913): 833. Samuel Dixon announced that researchers at the Pennsylvania state laboratory had inoculated a monkey with the polio virus by a fly bite, injected infected material into a second monkey, and thereby proven the fly a carrier; *Evening Bulletin,* August 30, 1916.

116. Telegram from Emerson to Felt, August 5, 1916, BO572, Box 26, New York State Archives. Felt suggested that Emerson hire entomologist R[alph] R[obinson] Parker of Powderville, Montana; Felt to Emerson, August 7, 1916, BO572, Box 26, New York State Archives. Parker was engaged in research on Rocky Mountain spotted fever.

117. Felt to Biggs, August 14, 1916, BO572, Box 25, New York State Archives. "These latter may play a minor or a major part in the dissemination of this plague and in view of the vital importance of the problem, it is obvious that no stone should be left unturned in a serious effort to limit this disease."

118. Ibid.

119. *New York Times,* August 11, 1916.

120. C. T. Brues, *Insects as Possible Carriers of Poliomyelitis Infection* (New York: Department of Health, no. 60, July 1917), 21–22, 4.

121. Ibid., 28, 29.

122. The pamphlet, published in 1917, was part of Emerson's *Monograph* of the 1916 epidemic. See ibid., 26: "To deny that animal reservoirs exist is taking much for granted, particularly as it is very probable than even in children a large number of abortive non-paralytic cases occur. That such cases should be the prevalent type in some animal acting as a reservoir is at least perfectly plausible."

123. *Evening Bulletin,* July 26, 1916. See also Simon Flexner and Paul F. Clark, "Contamination of the Fly with Poliomyelitis Virus," *JAMA* 56 (1911): 1717–1718.

124. *Philadelphia Inquirer,* August 5, 1916; *Newark Evening News,* July 5, 1916. Dixon also required all manure to be removed from stables at least twice a week during the fly season.

125. *Newark Evening News,* July 22, 1916. On the anti-fly campaign in Newark, see Stuart Galishoff, "Newark and the Great Polio Epidemic of 1916," *New Jersey History* 54 (1976): 106.

126. *New York Times,* August 18, 1916.

127. New York residents of Washington Heights swatted flies clad in Palm Beach suits, flannel trousers, and "other summer garb"; *New York Times,* July 9, 1916; *Philadelphia Inquirer,* July 27, 1916.

128. *New York Times,* July 23, 1916; *Evening Bulletin,* July 6, 1916.

129. *Newark Evening News,* June 12, 1916.

130. *New York Times,* July 13, 1916.

131. *Philadelphia Inquirer,* August 14, 1916.

132. *Evening Bulletin,* August 4, 1916.

133. *Philadelphia Inquirer,* August 5, 1916. The Staten Island group announced that the treatment of garbage on the island was probably responsible for the spread of polio, as flies attracted to the refuse carried the disease to nearby communities; *New York Times,* July 7, 1916.

134. *New York Times,* July 5, 1916; "A Mother," letter to editor, *Evening Bulletin,* September 16, 1916. See also Galishoff, "Great Polio Epidemic," 101–111. Some writers were even critical of specific methods. In a letter to a Philadelphia newspaper, one man criticized the proposed use of mosquito netting to protect food in city markets. "It is hard to understand what manner of germ will be kept out by a mesh of twelve holes to the inch"; S. S. Graves, letter to editor, *Evening Bulletin,* September 14, 1916.

135. Editorial, *New York Times,* July 13, 1916; letter to Mayor Mitchel, General Correspondence 1916, Municipal Archives, New York City.

136. *Evening Bulletin,* August 1, 1916.

137. Ibid. One writer warned that "the inspectors he [Krusen] appoints will be handy at the next election, and there is a lot of graft to it"; F. H., letter to editor, *Evening Bulletin,* August 22, 1916.

138. *Newark Evening News,* July 11, 1916. For a similar story about flies and a dead cat, see editorial, "State Boards Hands Off," *Newark Evening News,* July 12, 1916; and editorial, "Dead Animals in the Streets," *Newark Evening News,* July 13, 1916.

139. *Philadelphia Inquirer,* August 15, 1916; *Evening Bulletin,* July 24, 1916; *New York Times,* July 25, 1916; *Newark Evening News,* July 20, 1916. See also Hoy, " 'Municipal Housekeeping,' " 173–198.

140. Haven Emerson to Simon Flexner, September 21, 1916, Emerson file, Flexner papers, APS.

CHAPTER 3. THE PROMISE OF SCIENCE

1. John Ashburton Cutter [secretary, West Side Physicians Economic League] to E. P. Felt [New York State entomologist], November 9, 1916, BO572 Box 25, New York State Archives, Albany, New York.

2. George C. Slattery, "Newer Methods of Diagnosis," *American Medicine* 11 (1916): 312. "Clinicians must be developed as in the past," he argued, but added that the experimenter "is our future," 312.

3. Thomas Dixon [Brooklyn oculist] to Mitchel, July 13, 1916, General correspondence 1916, Municipal Archives, New York City.

4. Rosenberg, *The Care of Strangers,* 190–211.

5. See Maulitz, "Physician Versus Bacteriologist," 91–107; Morman, "Clinical Pathology in America," 198–214; Starr, *Social Transformation,* 145–179; and Kenneth M. Ludmerer, *Learning to Heal: The Development of American Medical Education* (New York: Basic Books, 1985), 207–218.

6. G. A. Ehret [Cleveland, Ohio], for example, used stock vaccines for pneumonia, gonorrhea, bronchial asthma, and rheumatism; "Vaccine Therapy," *Medical Record* 89 (1916): 328–329. On stock and autogeneous vaccines, see William Hallock Park and Anna Wessels Williams, assisted by Charles Krumwiede, Jr., *Pathogenic Microorganisms: A Practical Manual for Students, Physicians and Health Officers* 6th ed. (New York: Lea & Febiger, 1914), 585, 590.

7. F. Robbins, "Fifty Years of Medical Progress," *Medical Record* 89 (1916): 429.

8. Francis C. Peabody, George Draper, and A. R. Dochez, *A Clinical Study of Acute Poliomyelitis* (New York: Rockefeller Institute of Medical Research, no. 4, June 1, 1912), 7, 14. See also Paul, *History,* 118–123, 252–254; Saul Benison, "Speculation and Experimentation in Early Poliomyelitis Research," *Clio Medica* 10 (1975): 1–22. Polio was one of five diseases chosen for special study at the hospital; and Rufus Cole, head of the hospital, had high hopes for this polio study, for "it seemed to present exactly the kind of problems The

Rockefeller Institute was prepared to deal with effectively." See Corner, *Rockefeller Institute*, 98, 104, 106. Draper and Dochez went later to Columbia and Peabody to Harvard.

9. Peabody, Draper, and Dochez, *Study*, 19, 26. In 1912 the authors acknowledged that the appearance of paralysis did not equal polio, for its prominence in diagnosis might be "dependent in large part on our imperfect methods" (56).

10. Ibid., 33, 38–39, 46, 95–97, 98–107, 117.

11. Paul, *History*, 120–123. For one study contrasting clinical to experimental work, see Le G. Kerr, "Acute Anterior Poliomyelitis," *Long Island Medical Journal* (1909); abstract, *JAMA* 53 (1909): 1945.

12. See Corner, *Rockefeller Institute;* Benison, "Speculation"; and Benison, *Rivers.*

13. This belief was also evident to some extent in the laboratory work pursued by health officials in the New York City Health Department's Bureau of Laboratories, in state-funded laboratories in New York, Vermont, Massachusetts, and Pennsylvania, and by federal researchers at the Public Health Service's Hygienic Laboratory in Washington, D.C.

14 See Ivar Wickman, *Acute Poliomyelitis (Heine-Medin's Disease),* translated by J.W.A.W. Maloney (1907; New York: Journal of Nervous and Mental Disease, no. 16, 1913); Paul H. Roemer, *Epidemic Infantile Paralysis (Heine-Medin Disease),* translated by H. Ridley Prentice (1911; London: John Bale, Sons & Daniellson, 1913). In 1910 a New York neurologist urged his colleagues to learn to diagnose polio early, "a task more difficult than the interpretation of the so-called atypical cases"; Joseph Collins, "The Epidemiology of Poliomyelitis: A Plea That It May Be Considered a Reportable Disease," *JAMA* 54 (1910): 1928.

15. "The gross manifestations, as we know it, is a myelitis; but all the recent evidences show that we are dealing with a general intoxication, an infection of some sort"; Arthur S. Hamilton, [Minneapolis], "Discussion [of Treatment of Infantile Paralysis]," *JAMA* 55 (1910): 1020.

16. See, for example, Brandt, *No Magic Bullet;* Daniel M. Fox, "Social Policy and City Politics: Tuberculosis Reporting in New York, 1889–1900," *Bulletin of the History of Medicine* 49 (1975): 169–175; and Elizabeth Fee and Daniel M. Fox, eds., *AIDS: The Burdens of History* (Berkeley: University of California Press, 1988).

17. The Rockefeller researchers' list of the various diagnoses for polio cases that had ended up at the Rockefeller Institute's Hospital included tonsillitis, malaria, and pneumonia; Peabody, Draper, and Dochez, *Study*, 38; for a similar list see also W. H. Frost to Surgeon-General, October 25, 1911, Record Group 90-1712, Box 157, National Archives. Of sixty-three children sent by the New York City Department of Health to a city hospital during the summer of 1916, four had rickets and meningitis, and one was not sick; Walter Lester

Carr, "A Contribution on Poliomyelitis," *Transactions of American Pediatric Society* 29 (1917): 240.

18. H. W. Hill to Flexner, November 16, 1909, Polio file, Flexner papers, APS. For doctors who refused to report polio cases to state health authorities, see "Minutes," September 5, 1916, Health Department of the State of New Jersey, New Jersey State Archives, Trenton, New Jersey.

19. W. H. Frost to Surgeon-General, October 25, 1911, Cincinnati, Ohio, Record Group 90-1712, Box 157, National Archives.

20. See, for example, John Lovett Morse, "Infantile Paralysis: Spinal Form," *American Journal of Diseases of Children* 2 (1911): 94–95.

21. Emerson, *Monograph*, 90.

22. See Fox, "Social Policy and City Politics"; and Duffy, *Public Health in New York City*, 103–104.

23. A Philadelphia physician, W. Schler Bryant, was not convinced that polio germs did enter the blood stream, for, he argued, all known germs develop antibodies; but there were none known for polio; *New York Times*, July 10, 1916. This also meant that there could be no possible antitoxin.

24. One physician suggested fifteen cubic centimeters every twenty to twenty-four hours; Abraham Zingher, "The Diagnosis and Serum Treatment of Anterior Poliomyelitis," *JAMA* 68 (1917): 818. "No laboratory diagnostic methods of demonstrated reliability and universal application have been evolved. The early examination of cerbrospinal fluid is the most reliable laboratory method at present known"; John F. Anderson and Wade H. Frost, "Abortive Cases of Poliomyelitis: An Experimental Demonstration of Specific Immune Bodies in their Blood-Serum," *JAMA* 56 (1911): 667.

25. L. Emmett Holt, "Observations of Three Hundred Cases of Acute Meningitis in Infants and Young Children," *American Journal of Diseases of Children* 1 (1911): 26–36.

26. *Infantile Paralysis Committee Report* ([New York]: n. p., May 1917), 5.

27. Anderson and Frost, "Abortive Cases of Poliomyelitis," 667.

28. Phebe L. DuBois and Josephine B. Neal, "Summary of Four Years of Clinical and Bacteriological Experience with Meningitis in New York City," *American Journal of Diseases of Children* 9 (1915): 1–2.

29. Simon Flexner developed both a diagnostic test for meningcoccus in the spinal fluid and an anti-meningitis serum; Corner, *Rockefeller Institute*, 56–60. His work was so successful that a few years later the New York City Health Department took over the meningitis research and established a meningitis division of the Bureau of Laboratories. By 1916 this division employed a number of skilled pathologists who had the interest and ability to undertake research on polio as well.

30. John Randolph Graham, "The Poliomyelitis Epidemic—A Review of the Field Work Performed by the Health Department," *American Medicine* 11 (1916): 832–833.

31. Harry L. Abramson, "Discussion" of Wardner D. Ayer, "The Early Diagnosis of Poliomyelitis," *New York State Journal of Medicine* 17 (1917): 373.

32. New York health official William H. Park was not convinced that the only way to identify a polio case was to inject monkeys with washings of the patient's mucous membranes, for, he argued, most washings fail; "Infantile Paralysis: A Round Table Discussion," *American Journal of Public Health* 7 (1917): 134; hereafter cited "Round Table." Park admitted that spinal fluid analysis might be helpful in diagnosing doubtful cases, "but the findings in themselves never give us the information to make the absolute diagnosis of poliomyelitis" for there was no way to detect specific bacteria as in meningitis and tubercular meningitis; "Round Table," 138, 139.

33. Paul, *History*, 153, 156. Flexner doubted that the virus could be seen under an ordinary microscope, although he referred to having seen minute circular or slightly oval points in the dark microscope; *New York Times Magazine*, July 9, 1916. By 1908 about thirty organisms had been reported; see Robert W. Lovett and W. P. Lucas, "Infantile Paralysis: A Study of 635 Cases from the Children's Hospital, Boston, with Especial Reference to Treatment," *JAMA* 51 (1908): 1678.

34. A. L. Skoog, "Discussion [of Treatment of Infantile Paralysis]," *JAMA* 55 (1910): 1019. On the use of complement binding experiments with fluid and blood serum, see also M. Allen Starr, "Epidemic Infantile Paralysis [and] Discussion," *JAMA* 51 (1908): 112–113.

35. See Editorial, "Bacteriology of Poliomyelitis," *JAMA* 68 (1917): 1122–1123.

36. Zingher, "Diagnosis and Serum," 817–818.

37. During a polio outbreak in Billings, Montana, A. J. Lanza, a federal health service official, disproved the diagnosis of a local physician who had claimed a patient had epidemic cerebrospinal meningitis. "A spinal puncture was made in my presence," Lanza reported, "also a puncture of the lateral ventricle, and the fluid was clear and watery and microscopic examinations showed no evidence of meningitis"; A. J. Lanza to Surgeon-General, August 23, 1916, Record Group 90-1712, Box 157, National Archives.

38. All that was available were "simple chemical and cytological tests"; Peabody, Draper, and Dochez, *Study*, 99.

39. DuBois and Neal, "Meningitis," 3.

40. One physician noted that the changes in the spinal fluid were not characteristic of the disease alone, but they were useful in differentiating the disease: increased cell count, globulin content, increased lymphocytes,

and the fact that no [bacterial] organisms could be cultivated. Francis R. Fraser, "Epidemic Poliomyelitis: Symptomatology and Diagnosis in the Acute Stages," *Boston Medical and Surgical Journal* (1916); abstract, *Pediatrics* 28 (1916): 472–473. Fraser studied 126 cases of polio patients' spinal fluid noting changes in the number of cells, the extent of globulin present, and the ability to reduce Fehling's solution. Fraser, "Study of Cerebrospinal Fluid in Acute Poliomyelitis," *Journal of Experimental Medicine* (1913); abstract, *JAMA* 61 (1913): 992–993.

41. H. L. Abramson, "The Spinal Fluid in Poliomyelitis and its Differentiation from Fluids of Other Infections," *American Journal of Diseases of Children* 10 (1915): 345–348. Abramson had discovered some unusually large mononuclear cells, which, he hazarded, might offer polio researchers a more definite way of differentiating between polio and meningitis cases.

42. Ibid., 348. Federal officials argued that "total and differential leukocyte counts offer a promising aid to diagnosis, but much more work will be necessary to establish the reliability of this method"; "until the clinical recognition of poliomyelitis is placed on a more reliable basis there will remain an indeterminable factor in its epidemiology," and conclusions from epidemiological data "will have to be correspondingly conservative." Anderson and Frost, "Abortive Cases of Poliomyelitis," 667.

43. Edward E. Mayer, letter to editor, *JAMA* 55 (1910): 1397; and Mayer to Flexner, September 24, 1910, Polio file, Flexner papers, APS.

44. DuBois and Neal, "Meningitis," 5; see also Josephine Neal and Phoebe DuBois, "The Diagnosis of Poliomyelitis," *American Journal of Medical Sciences* 512 (1916): 318–319.

45. Abramson, "Discussion," 373.

46. F.W.C. Mohr to Flexner, August 17, 1910; Flexner to Mohr [copy], August 29, 1910; Mohr to Flexner, September 4, 1910, Polio file, Flexner papers, APS. According to Zingher, anesthesia was generally unnecessary unless the child struggled; "Diagnosis and Serum," 818.

47. Edward E. Mayer, letter to editor, *JAMA* 55 (1910): 1396–1397; Mayer to Flexner, September 24, 1910, Polio file, Flexner papers, APS.

48. Flexner, letter to editor, *JAMA* 55 (1910): 1397; Flexner to Mayer, October 1, 1910, Polio file, Flexner papers, APS. See also Theo. Colman to Flexner, August 23, 1910, Polio file, Flexner papers, APS.

49. Flexner to Mayer, October 1, 1910, Polio file, Flexner papers, APS.

50. Theo. Colman to Flexner, August 23, 1910, Polio file, Flexner papers, APS.

51. DuBois and Neal, "Meningitis," 1.

52. Paul A. Lewis to Flexner, August 17, 1910, Polio file, Flexner papers, APS.

53. At one city hospital physicians performed 250 lumbar punctures on sixty-three children; Carr, "A Contribution," 244.

54. Holt, "Observations," 26, 27, 36.

55. Lewis F. Frissell, "Report of a Case of Epidemic Anterior Poliomyelitis: Diagnosis in Preparalytic Stage by Lumbar Puncture," *JAMA* 56 (1911): 661–662.

56. Holt, "Observations," 31, 35.

57. Paul, *History*, chaps. 4–12.

58. George H. Simmons to Flexner, September 8, 1910, Polio file, Flexner papers, APS; Flexner did suggest that hexamethylenamin had a "high degree of antiseptic action." "Infantile Paralysis a Scourge and Puzzle," *New York Times Magazine*, July 9, 1916.

59. Abraham Sophian, "Specific Treatment of Infantile Paralysis: Preliminary Note," *JAMA* 67 (1916): 426–427.

60. See John Harley Warner, *The Therapeutic Perspective: Medical Practice, Knowledge and Identity in America, 1820–1885* (Cambridge: Harvard University Press, 1986).

61. Frissell, "Report of a Case," 662. Many patients derived relief from mild mustard plasters to the spine; W. House, "Acute Anterior Poliomyelitis," *Northwest Medicine*, (1910); abstract, *JAMA* 55 (1910): 1411.

62. Phillip F. Barbour, "Epidemic Anterior Poliomyelitis," abstract, *JAMA* 61 (1913): 988.

63. *Medical Record* 98 (1916): 40.

64. "Discussion on Symposium on Poliomyelitis," *Transactions of American Pediatric Society* 23 (1911): 225. Samuel Gross in a 1872 lecture suggested bleeding, blisters, and mercury ointment; cited in Paul, *History*, 62–65. In the second edition of Michael Underwood's *Diseases of Children* (1789), which provided the first clinical description of the disease, the author suggested the use of cathartics, blisters, purgatives, emetics, and electricity; Paul, *History*, 23. The first American edition of Underwood in 1818 also stressed bloodletting; Paul, *History*, 36.

65. H. M. McClanahan, "Treatment of the Acute Stage," *JAMA* 55 (1910): 1464.

66. C. E. Dakin, "Acute Epidemic Poliomyelitis," *Iowa Medical Journal* (1910); abstract, *JAMA* 55 (1910): 2097; see also Lovett and Lucas, "Infantile Paralysis," 1681.

67. On applying "general symptomatic procedures," see Peabody, Draper, and Dochez, *Study*, 115.

68. Kerr, "Acute," 1945.

69. M. Neustaedter, "The Diagnosis and Treatment of Acute Anterior Poliomyelitis in the Preparalytic and Postparalytic Stages," *New York Medical Journal* 54 (1916): 145, 146, 148. Hermann Biggs, head of New York State's Board of Health, suggested, if necessary, a drop of "deodorized tincture of opium every hour until quieted"; *New York Times,* July 7, 1916. A physician from Portland, Oregon, suggested using bromides and codeine and perhaps atropine and inhalations of oxygen if there were respiratory problems; House, "Acute Anterior Poliomyelitis," 1411.

70. Carr, "A Contribution," 244, 246.

71. Barbour, "Epidemic Anterior Poliomyelitis," 988. But a Kentucky physician felt that strychnine was as dangerous as alcohol; its continued use "will invariably do harm," for polio was "a disease of impaired nutrition." Instead doctors needed to equalize their patients' blood pressure by systematic rest, the proper application of hydrotherapy, elimination, and "not too active catharsis"; "Discussion" at Kentucky Medical Association Annual Meeting, *JAMA* 61 (1913): 988.

72. Kentucky Medical Association, "Discussion," 988.

73. McClanahan, "Treatment," 1464.

74. Osler, *Practice of Medicine,* cited in Paul, *History,* 70.

75. Lovett and Lucas, "Infantile Paralysis," 1681.

76. B. Sachs, "Treatment from the Neurologist's Viewpoint," *JAMA* 55 (1910): 1465. Bernard Sachs, a New York neurologist, had headed the 1907 Investigation Committee of the New York City polio epidemic.

77. S. J. Crowe, "The Excretion of Hexamethylenamin (Urotropin) in the Cerebrospinal Fluid and Its Therapeutic Value in Meningitis," *Bulletin of Johns Hopkins Hospital* 20 (1909): 102–105. See also Charles Herrman, "The Communicability of Acute Poliomyelitis: Its Spread and Control," *American Medicine* 11 (1916): 713–720; and E. H. Bradford, R. W. Lovett, et al., "Methods of Treatment in Infantile Paralysis," in *Infantile Paralysis in Massachusetts in 1909* (Boston: Wright & Potter, 1910), 69–98.

78. Collins, "The Epidemiology of Poliomyelitis," 1928.

79. In 1911, a California doctor reported he had been prescribing hexamethylenamin for the past year as a remedy for common colds, influenced by the work of Crowe and Cushing: "As a cure for colds it may be as great a boon as it has been proved to be as a urinary antiseptic"; Austin Miller, "Hexamethylenamin: A Remedy for Common Colds," *JAMA* 56 (1910): 1718. On its use for pellagra, see Walter E. Vest, letter to editor, *JAMA* 55 (1910): 1828.

80. Frissell, "Report of a Case," 662. The California State Board of Medical Examiners suggested using two or three grains of urotropin every two hours during acute stages; *Medical Record* 89 (1916): 393; and see also McClanahan, "Treatment of the Acute Stage," 1464. A Kentucky physician used hexamethylenamin in early cases of polio "with excellent results"; Ken-

tucky Medical Association, "Discussion," 988. Starr mentioned Cushing's work on urotropin in cerebral surgery and suggested using it for nervous diseases where an infection was suspected; "Epidemic Infantile Paralysis," 118.

81. Robert B. Preble, letter to editor, *JAMA* 55 (1910): 1130. Skoog used about three grams a day; "Treatment," 1804.

82. H. W. Hill to Flexner, July 5, 1911, Polio file, Flexner papers, APS. For the use of urotropin as therapy for Rocky Mountain spotted fever, see Victoria A. Harden, *Rocky Mountain Spotted Fever: History of a Twentieth-Century Disease* (Baltimore: Johns Hopkins University Press, 1990), 198.

83. Flexner and Lewis, "Seventh Note," 1782.

84. Frissell, "Report of a Case," 662. Neustaedter urged nasal spray of hydrogen peroxide, as well as disinfectants for all discharges; Neustaedter, "Diagnosis and Treatment," 148.

85. Beverly Robinson, "Infantile Paralysis," *New York Medical Journal* 54 (1916): 128.

86. "Discussion," *Journal of Electrotherapeutics and Radiology* 34 (1916): 518–519.

87. For support of lumbar puncture for both diagnosis and treatment, see Andrew L. Skoog [Kansas neurologist], "Treatment of Acute Anterior Polio myelitis," *JAMA* 55 (1910): 1804.

88. DuBois and Neal, "Meningitis," 7; Abramson, "Spinal Fluid," 347; Abraham Sophian, "Specific Treatment of Infantile Paralysis: Preliminary Note," *JAMA* 67 (1916): 427. For work critical of lumbar puncture as therapy, see G. Canby Robinson, "The Blood-Pressure in Epidemic Cerebrospinal Meningitis," *Archives of Internal Medicine* 5 (1910): 488.

89. S. J. Meltzer, July 31, 1916, [copy of telegram], Polio correspondence, Administration, 301.2, Rockefeller Archive Center, Tarrytown, New York. See also A. McGehee Harvey, "Samuel J. Meltzer: Pioneer Catalyst in the Evolution of Clinical Science in America," *Perspectives in Biology and Medicine* 21 (1978): 431–440; and Corner, *Rockefeller Institute*, 117–120.

90. Editorial, *New York Medical Journal* 104 (1916): 221. Physicians and the public needed a more rigorous explanation of the therapy than phrases such as "a wonderful tonic," "removes pressure from nervous tissues," and "places nature in a position to do the rest." A New York physician argued against the use of both the lumbar puncture and adrenalin after his experience with one case. He had made a puncture and withdrew ten cubic centimeters of fluid, then injected two cubic centimeters of adrenalin, giving four injections in all. His patient gradually grew worse and died. "The lesson was learned"; J. Gardner Smith, "Discussion," *Journal of Electrotherapeutics and Radiology* 34 (1916): 523–524. Emerson admitted that adrenalin therapy was not being carried out fully as doctors in charge "could not convince themselves that they

get [got] relief or promising results"; "Conference of Infantile Paralysis held at the office of [the] Rockefeller Foundation, Saturday, August 5, 1916, 10 o'clock A. M.," Flexner papers, #200/25/283, Rockefeller Archive Center, Tarrytown, New York, 14.

91. *New York Times,* August 10, 1916.

92. Editorial, "Their Help Has Not Been Great," *New York Times,* August 8, 1916. Emerson defended Meltzer's exclusion by arguing that the conference had included only bacteriologists and Meltzer was a physiologist; *New York Times,* August 3, 1916.

93. Anderson and Frost, "Abortive Cases," 666.

94. Flexner, letter to editor, *JAMA* 55 (1910): 1397; Flexner, letter to *JAMA* editor, October 1, 1910, Polio files, Flexner papers, APS. On the logic of using a drug that aided one disease for another disease with similar symptoms, see Harden, *Spotted Fever,* 199. On the importance of the anti-meningitis serum for establishing support for the Rockefeller Institute, see Saul Benison, "The History of Polio Research in the United States: Appraisal and Lessons," in Gerald Holton, ed., *The Twentieth Century Sciences: Studies in the Biography of Ideas* (New York: W. W. Norton, 1972), 315.

95. Duffy, *Public Health in New York City,* chap. 11; Bushel, *Chronology of New York City Department of Health.*

96. Duffy, *Public Health in New York City,* 99–102.

97. *Philadelphia Inquirer,* August 27, 1916.

98. As cited by H. W. Frauenthal, "The Treatment of Infantile Paralysis Based on the Present Epidemic," *Journal of Electrotherapeutics and Radiology* 34 (1916): 506. He noted that polio's microorganism had not yet been detected in the circulating blood, 506.

99. Paul, *History,* 190–194. Trials of this sera in the 1930s were not conclusive; Paul, *History,* 390; Harry F. Dowling, *Fighting Infection: Conquests of the Twentieth Century* (Cambridge: Harvard University Press, 1977), 206.

100. Editorial, *JAMA* 61 (1913): 1904–1905. Flexner argued that polio serum sometimes but not always helped avert paralysis, "Infantile Paralysis a Scourge and Puzzle," *New York Times Magazine,* July 9, 1916.

101. Neal and DuBois, "Poliomyelitis," 315.

102. Anderson and Frost, "Abortive Cases of Poliomyelitis," 988. Flexner and Lewis's experiments with recovered serum also proved successful. "The successful outcome of this experiment suggested that the blood of persons who had recovered from poliomyelitis contained similar immunity principles." They used children's blood serum successfully but not horse serum, which they found tended to hasten the onset of paralysis; Simon Flexner and Paul A. Lewis, "Experimental Poliomyelitis in Monkeys: Seventh Note: Active Immunization and Passive Serum Protection," *JAMA* 54 (1910): 1780–1782. Note that this interest in the antibody properties of the blood of polio patients

did not alter the accepted model of the polio virus traveling through nervous tissues.

103. G. A. Rueck, "Three Cases of Acute Anterior Poliomyelitis Treated Successfully by Transfusion of Citrated Normal Blood of Adults," *Medical Record* 90 (1916): 587.

104. Paul, *History,* 190–197.

105. *New York Times,* July 17, August 13, August 15, 1916; *Evening Bulletin,* August 21, 1916; and see Paul, *History,* 192–193. A federal health official used lumbar puncture with cell count and Noguchi's globulin test for diagnosis. If it proved positive but the case had no paralysis, he used serum treatment "with apparently excellent results"; L. Fricks to Surgeon-General, October 17, 1916, Record Group 90-1712, Box 157, National Archives, Washington, D.C.

106. *Evening Bulletin,* August 29, 1916; *Philadelphia Inquirer,* August 15, 1916. In New York a citizen's committee was formed to get an added supply of immune serum from the 700 or so people known to have recovered from the disease; *Medical Record,* 90 (1916): 376.

107. *New York Times,* August 2, August 16, 1916. He believed that it had beneficial results, both when injected subcutaneously and intramuscularly; *Philadelphia Inquirer,* August 10, 1916. Emerson reported that immune serum had been used with some good results in twenty to thirty cases at city hospitals and by various doctors. It was used almost exclusively in very severe cases or at early onset of paralysis; "Rockefeller Conference," 14.

108. Neustaedter, "Diagnosis and Treatment," 147. But he felt that a vaccine based on an attenuated virus was more promising than recovered serum.

109. Emerson, *Monograph,* 286.

110. *New York Times,* August 9, 1916. Philadelphia police surgeons requested members of the force to donate their blood; *Evening Bulletin,* August 29, 1916.

111. Frederick T. H. to Flexner, August 29, 1916, Polio file, Flexner papers, APS.

112. Mrs. F. D. D. [Escanaba, Michigan] to Flexner, August 22, 1910, Polio file, Flexner papers, APS.

113. Charles H. [Middletown, Connecticut] to Flexner, October 12, 1910, Polio file, Flexner papers, APS. A "very important family," "one of the Rockefeller connections," wanted to protect a child from the possibility of polio and needed a doctor to administer serum; Simon Flexner to Francis W. Peabody [Peter Bent Brigham Hospital, Boston], May 12, 1917, Polio file, Flexner Papers, APS. In a private meeting George Draper admitted that to meet the sudden appearance of cases "the puncture is made, and it is a kind of a hurry up, and there is not time to do a Wassermann"; "Rockefeller Conference," 64.

114. Edmond J. Melville, "The Physician of Yesterday," *American Medicine* 11 (1916): 586.

115.   Anonymous, "Report Division of Pathology and Bacteriology, 1915," 8, Record Group 90-5016, National Archives. The Hygienic Laboratory author found the charge "extremely improbable." Compare Judith Walzer Leavitt, "Politics and Public Health: Smallpox in Milwaukee, 1894–1895," *Bulletin of the History of Medicine* 50 (1976): 553–568.

116.   Eugene Barton, letter to editor, *Evening Bulletin*, August 25, 1916.

CHAPTER 4. WRITTEN IN HASTE
1.   Mrs. C. M., August 4, 1916, Box C #7, Polio file, Flexner papers, APS, Philadelphia, Pennsylvania; hereafter cited Polio APS. All last names will be identified by initial only.

2.   Mrs. L. B., September 15, 1916, Box C #8, Polio APS. Letters to Mayor John Mitchel can be found in his papers, General Correspondence, 1916, #1712, Boxes A to W, New York City Municipal Archives; hereafter cited Mitchell NYC. Letters to the New York City's Health Department are discussed in Emerson, *Monograph*, 75–77. Emerson stated that his department had received 230 letters, but he provided little information about their authors. Letters were also published in local newspapers, but even during the peak of the 1916 epidemic most daily city papers, such as the *New York Times*, the *Philadelphia Inquirer*, and the *Newark Evening News*, printed only about four letters a week. Jessie P., an attorney, told Mitchel that he had gone to the *New York Times* offices and been told that reporters were "in receipt of thousands of letters, but were not allowed to publish anything in regard to the paralysis epidemic which would be exciting"; August 3, 1916, Mitchel NYC.

3.   Roy Porter, "Introduction," *Patients and Practitioners: Lay Perceptions of Medicine in Pre-Industrial Society*, ed. Roy Porter (Cambridge: Cambridge University Press, 1985), 3. See also Porter, "The Patient's View: Doing Medical History from Below," *Theory and Society* 14 (1985): 175–198.

4.   See, for example, Michael MacDonald, *Mystical Bedlam: Madness, Anxiety, and Healing in Seventeenth-Century England* (Cambridge: Cambridge University Press, 1981); Charles E. Rosenberg, "The Therapeutic Revolution: Medicine, Meaning and Social Change in Nineteenth-Century America," in *The Therapeutic Revolution: Essays in the Social History of Medicine*, ed. Morris J. Vogel and Rosenberg (Philadelphia: University of Pennsylvania Press, 1979), 3–25; Rosenberg, "Medical Text and Social Context: Explaining William Buchan's *Domestic Medicine*," *Bulletin of the History of Medicine* 57 (1983): 22–42; Steven Feierman, "The Struggle for Control: The Social Roots of Health and Healing in Modern Africa," *African Studies Review* 28 (1985): 73–85; Andrew Weir, "Puritan Perceptions of Illness of Seventeenth-Century England," in *Patients and Practitioners*, 55–99; and Lucinda McCray Beier, *Sufferers and Healers: The Experience of Illness in Seventeenth-Century England* (London: Routledge and Kegan Paul, 1987).

5. Judith Walzer Leavitt, *Brought to Bed: Childbearing in America, 1750–1950* (New York: Oxford University Press, 1986); and Rima D. Apple, *Mothers and Medicine: A Social History of Infant Feeding, 1890–1950* (Madison: University of Wisconsin Press, 1987).

6. Maurice M. M., August 10, 1916, Box C #7, Polio APS.

7. Emerson, *Monograph*, 75.

8. Benison, *Rivers*, 128.

9. The 161 letters from the Flexner collection that can be definitely identified: New England, 14; Mid-Atlantic, 91; Midwest, 22; South, 10; West and Southwest, 15; Canada, 8; Australia, 1. The twenty-two letters in the Mitchel collection are similarly distributed: Manhattan, 9; Brooklyn, 3; New York area, 5; South, 4; California, 1.

10. Leila L., August 12, 1916, Box C #10, Polio APS. Of 168 letters from the Flexner collection in which gender can be definitely identified, eighty-two were written by men and eighty-six by women. All twenty-two letters I found addressed to Mitchel were written by men, often as representatives of political or social organizations.

11. Mrs. A.E.W., September 17, 1916, Box C #9, Polio APS.

12. Daniel R. J., September [n. d.] 1916, Box C #5, Polio APS; Caesar R., July 11, 1916, Box C #4, Polio APS; Samuel K., July 6, 1916, Box C #4, Polio APS.

13. Mrs W. H., August 23, 1916, Box C #1, Polio APS.

14. N.M.W., November 24, 1916, Box C #8, Polio APS.

15. Edward H. O., December 8, 1916, Box C #3, Polio APS.

16. C.E.B., August 24, 1916, Box C #5, Polio APS.

17. *New York Times*, July 16, 1916; July 12, 1916. Richard T. Crane, Jr., of Chicago also offered $25,000 for the "best cure" of polio; *New York Times*, August 9, 1916.

18. Orville M. K., September 23, 1916, Box C #9, Polio APS.

19. Emerson, *Monograph*, 76; see also *Philadelphia Inquirer*, August 5, 1916.

20. Hughes B. W., July 17, 1916, Box C #8, Polio APS. For additional work on domestic medicine and lay therapy, see Rosenberg, "The Therapeutic Revolution"; John B. Blake, "From Buchan to Fishbein: The Literature of Domestic Medicine," in *Medicine Without Doctors: Home Health Care in American History*, ed. Guenter B. Risse, Ronald L. Numbers, and Judith Walzer Leavitt (New York: Science History, 1977), 11–30; and James T. Patterson, *The Dread Disease: Cancer and Modern American Culture* (Cambridge: Harvard University Press, 1987), 231–240.

21. Mrs. V.C.Y., August 8, 1916, Box C #2, Polio APS; H.C.A.F., July 19, 1916, Mitchel NYC.

22. C.L.M., August 4, 1916, Box C #7, Polio APS; Mrs. Addie S., August 8, 1916, Box C #6, Polio APS.

23. *Newark Evening News,* July 8, 1916. See also Rosenberg, *The Cholera Years,* 22.

24. See, for example, Priscilla E. G., August 6, 1916, Box C #3, Polio APS.

25. Edward H. O., July 25, 1916, Box C #3; Edward H. O., August 9, 1916, Box C #3, Polio APS.

26. Mrs. T., September 18, 1916, Box C #9, Polio APS.

27. Katherine T., August 14, 1916, Box C #10, Polio APS. One man went so far as to invoke Tolstoy: Abraham Lebierkin, a Philadelphia tailor's assistant, who was reported to have a bottle of "white mixture" (a possible polio cure) made up by Ivan Ivanovich, Tolstoy's town chemist and apostle from Witekshi[?] in Russia; *Evening Bulletin,* August 10, 1916.

28. Mrs. Frances B., August 11, 1916, Box C #1, Polio APS.

29. E.G.B., August 3, 1916, Box C #6, Polio APS.

30. Captain John S. T., August 16, 1916, Box C #1, Polio APS.

31. L.C.P., August 6, 1916, Box C #7, Polio APS; Margaret B. P., August 17, 1916, Box C #7, Polio APS.

32. The most detailed study of Thomsonians is still Alex Berman, "The Impact of the Nineteenth-Century Botanico-Medical Movement in American Pharmacy and Medicine" (Ph.D. diss., University of Wisconsin, 1954); and see also Berman, "The Thomsonian Movement and its Relation to American Pharmacy and Medicine," *Bulletin of the History of Medicine* 25 (1951): 405–428, 519–538.

33. L.C.P., ["Discoverer"], August 6, 1916, Box C #7, Polio APS.

34. J.E.H., October 4, 1916, Box C #5, Polio APS.

35. Mrs. Emma P. G., June 30, 1916, Box C #4, Polio APS.

36. J.W.D., September 4, 1916, Box C #5, Polio APS.

37. May W., August 8, 1916, Box C #7, Polio APS. She argued that her theory could explain why sanitary conditions did not appear relevant to the spread of polio and why most afflicted children had good or fair domestic hygiene.

38. J. F. van N., August 3, 1916, Box C #6, Polio APS.

39. "A Williamsburgh Pharmacist," August 9, 1916, Box C #7, Polio APS. For a suggestion of iodine injections used "intramuscularly," see David L., August 7, 1916, Box C #7, Polio APS; and see A. W., July 9, 1916, Box C #4, Polio APS.

40. Mrs. Fanny M. M., August 20, 1916, Box C #8, Polio APS; and see Emerson, *Monograph,* 76; Mrs. Nina H. P.-F., August 15, 1916, Box C #6, Polio APS.

41. William F. B., August 13, 1916, Box C #6, Polio APS.

42. Mrs. Nina H. P.-F., August 15, 1916, Box C #6, Polio APS; Walter J. F., August 6, 1916, Box C #7, Polio APS.

43. H.C.A.F., July 19, 1916, Mitchel NYC.

44. J. P. McR., July 14, 1916, Mitchel NYC; Hugh B. W., July 17, 1916, Box C #8, Polio APS.

45. Mrs. L. B., September 15, 1916, Box C #8, Polio APS; Mrs. M. R., August 29, 1916, Box C #5, Polio APS.

46. Thomas W., [November] 1916, Box C #8, Polio APS.

47. A.H.N., n.d., Box C #10, Polio APS. See James Harvey Young, *Pure Food: Securing the Federal Food and Drugs Act of 1906* (Princeton: Princeton University Press, 1989), 113–124.

48. Roderick T., August 9, 1916, Box C #6, Polio APS. See also E.P.V., July 8, 1916, Box C #4, Polio APS.

49. Emerson, *Monograph*, 76.

50. Mrs. M. R., August 29, 1916, Box C #5, Polio APS. The disinfectant, she explained, would rid sick bodies of thread worms, the cause, she believed, of numerous ills. She had given the remedy to her children and grandchildren "with wonderful results."

51. Priscilla E. G., August 6, 1916, Box C #3, Polio APS. Years earlier, she claimed, a doctor in her town had cured a child with infantile paralysis by using leeches.

52. See Rosenberg, "The Therapeutic Revolution."

53. Mrs. W., [August] 1916, Box C #6, Polio APS. See also G.Y.G., August 15, 1916, Mitchel NYC. This writer incorporated many of these methods into one list of "some methods of prevention for infantile paralysis" and sent it to the major of New York City. I quote the list:

1. Burning some tar and Camphor in living room.
2. Put some Limestone Chloride in toilet, around stable and in Ash can.
3. give Children camphor cigarett[e]s. . . .
5. Boiling milk which is sold 6 cents a quart.
6. put some garlick in the children[']s meals.

If you give these orders at once I am sure you [will] stop that disease in a short time.

54. Eugene C. G., August 10, 1916, Box C #6, Polio APS. On popular ideas for cancer therapy, see Patterson, *The Dread Disease*, 232–241.

55. "Washingtonian," August 16, 1916, Box C #7, Polio APS.

56. Emerson, *Monograph*, 76; Mrs. Addie S., August 8, 1916, Box C #6, Polio APS.

57. E.G.B., August 9, 1916, Box C #6, Polio APS; Mrs. W. H., August 29, 1916, Box C #1, Polio APS.

58. D.C.B., August 12, 1916, Box C #7, Polio APS; Mrs. Sara H. S., August 23, 1916, Box C #1, Polio APS.

59. Louise D. M., August 2, 1916, Box C #4, Polio APS.

60. F.J.S., August 17, 1916, Box C #7, Polio APS, warned that toxins from the bodies of fish were entering human stomachs and then the blood, thereby causing weakness and fever by "attacking Phagocytes." The antidote to fish poison was, he explained, prussic acid "very much attenuated." He also urged Flexner to try intramuscular iodine injections that were "useful in all bacterial invasions." See also David L., August 7, 1916, Box C #7, Polio APS.

61. David B. L., August 10, 1916, Box C #7, Polio APS. Inhaling iron fumes might cure "microscopic animals or germs, infesting the body," explained the Ohio iron worker, Daniel R. J., September 3, 1916, Box C #5, Polio APS.

62. Eucalyptus oil, when ingested, was so bitter that "no germ will live in its presence," wrote Patrick L. C.; it would cure polio, tuberculosis, and "any other germ disease"; Patrick L. C., September 26, 1916, Box C #8, Polio APS.

63. Mrs. Charles B. L., [August] 1916, Box C #10, Polio APS.

64. Archibald S., August 22, 1916, Box C #10, Polio APS; Arthur H. I., August 31, 1916, Box C #10, Polio APS.

65. See Leavitt, *The Healthiest City*, 180–189; Meckel, *Save the Babies*, chap. 3.

66. Mrs. E.V.T., [n.d.], Box C #7, Polio APS. See also Maurice M. M. who commented on the noticeable differences between pigs fed on whole milk and pasteurized milk, August 10, 1916, Box C #7, Polio APS.

67. Nathan Straus, October 19, 1916, Mitchel NYC; see also Straus to W. G. Simpson [acting surgeon-general] October 19, 1916, Record Group 90-1912, Box 157, National Archives, Washington, D.C.

68. Mrs. David H. D., August 5, 1916, Box C #2, Polio APS; Pauline M., [August] 1916, Box C #2, Polio APS.

69. Hannah A. G., August 9, 1916, Box C #6, Polio APS.

70. J.V.T., July 18, 1916, Mitchel NYC.

71. George B. C., July 11, 1916, Mitchel NYC; H.C.A.F., July 19, 1916, Mitchel NYC. Frank L. Donlus, president of the New York City Board of Aldermen, told the press that the epidemic would best be controlled not by "a crowd of medical diagnosticians from all over the country," but "a force of strong-armed men with shovels to rid our thousands of sewer-receiving basins of germ-laden refuse"; *New York Times*, July 29, 1916. On germs and moral randomness, see Rosenberg, "Florence Nightingale," 116–136.

72. Mrs. B. T., August 5, 1916, Box C #3, Polio APS.

73. See William F. B., August 13, 1916, Box C #6, Polio APS; H.C.A.F., July 19, 1916, Mitchel NYC. See also Andrew McClary, "Germs are Everywhere: The Germ Threat as Seen in Magazine Articles, 1890–1920," *Journal of American Culture* 3 (1980): 32–46.

74. Pauline M., [August] 1916, Box C #2, Polio APS. H. E., of Saratoga Springs, New York, felt that bottled milk and water should not be delivered to homes in infected areas; *New York Times*, August 14, 1916.

75. See Young, *Pure Food*, 106–113, 130–139, and chap. 10.

76. N.M.W., November 24, 1916, Box C #8, Polio APS.

77. Mrs. Walter G., August 16, 1916, Box C #1, Polio APS; Mrs. Ida M. S., August 31, 1916, Box C #5, Polio APS. For further analysis of women as domestic sanitarians and healers, see Hoy, " 'Municipal Housekeeping,' " 193–198.

78. Mrs. Lucy S. C., August 22, 1916, Box C #10, Polio APS. The cause, she argued, was not a germ but lead in flour. It was not strong enough to attack adults but was dangerous for children; and see Mrs. S.A.B., August 2, 1916, Box C #2, Polio APS.

79. Mrs. Minnie D. L., August 4, 1916, Box C #8, Polio APS. See also the danger of overripe bananas, "especially [from] the Italian fruit stands"; Grace F., August 18, 1916, Box C #9, Polio APS.

80. John K., August 28, 1916, Box C #10, Polio APS. On insects and disease, see Harden, *Spotted Fever;* and Rogers, "Germs with Legs," 599–617.

81. J. Hugo P., August 8, 1916, Box C #7, Polio APS.

82. This would explain unconnected and unexpected cases and the appearance of polio among children living in even the most careful and apparently sanitary conditions; Ida M. S., August 31, 1916, Box C #5, Polio APS.

83. Abrair S. K., August 30, 1916, Box C #5, Polio APS.

84. *Newark Evening News*, July 12, 1916. One man who sat in the park every day noticed that summer flies had a "strong, sharp and painful sting" and wondered if they might be the cause of the epidemic. He enclosed a few he had caught, noting that they were different from houseflies; M. R., [August] 1916, Box C #7, Polio APS. For an emphasis on fomites rather than flies, one woman blamed the epidemic on "Filthy Money," "which finds its way into all sorts of condition[s] in life. Think how money is handled, and by whom." "The public have [*sic*] a far more dangerous conveyer of germs than any flies." It could explain why Emerson had reported no case of polio among asylum children, as they did not handle money. Writing to the secretary of the treasury, she had suggested that money be cleaned before leaving the treasury "as it is a menace of life"; Mrs. J.T.C., August 27, 1916, Box C #8, Polio APS. See also Young to Young, August 14, 1916: Young reassured his wife that the letters he sent her written during the 1916 epidemic would not carry the disease.

85. W.L.D., August 24, 1916, Box C #5, Polio APS.

86. Alex C. T., September 11, 1916, Box C #7, Polio APS.

87. Mrs. Jeanette L., November 18, 1916, Box C #5, Polio APS.

88. H.M.B., August 8, 1916, Box C #2, Polio APS.

89. *Evening Bulletin,* September 11, 1916; *Philadelphia Inquirer,* July 20, 1916.

90. *Philadelphia Inquirer,* August 4, 1916.

91. "Skirts: The Shorter the Healthier: Science Now Vindicates the Abbreviated Costume," *Philadelphia Inquirer,* July 2, 1916.

92. On tuberculosis campaigns, see Dubos and Dubos, *The White Plague;* Michael E. Teller, *The Tuberculosis Movement: A Public Health Campaign in the Progressive Era* (Westport: Greenwood Press, 1988); and Feldberg, " 'An Antitoxin of Self-Respect.' "

93. "The Dean," September 16, 1916, Box C #8, Polio APS. Compare the warning of a physician who was widely quoted during the 1916 epidemic. He advised "a thorough scrubbing of the floors and frequent flushing of the streets and sidewalks . . . [for] we must remember that people spit on the sidewalks and children play there"; Neustaedter, "Diagnosis and Treatment," 148.

94. E.G.B., August 3, 1916, Box C #6, Polio APS.

95. Children were "especially susceptible in unhygienic surroundings"; Mrs. Minnie D. L., August 4, 1916, Box C #8, Polio APS.

96. See Rosenberg, "Medical Text and Social Context."

97. H.M.B., August 8, 1916, Box C #2, Polio APS.

98. Donald B. Armstrong, letter to editor, *New York Times,* July 19, 1916.

99. Mrs. Susan M. W., August 21, 1916, Box C #8, Polio APS; C.W.P., August 30, 1916, Box C #3, Polio APS.

100. Frank I. F., August 28, 1916, Box C #1, Polio APS; George W. W., August 9, 1916, Box C #2, Polio APS.

101. Percy E. W., August 21, 1916, Box C #10, Polio APS.

102. See Dr. W. H. Vail, "Till the Doctor Comes," on "Infantile Paralysis," *Newark Evening News,* July 12, 1916.

103. Frank R. S., August 29, 1916, Box C #10, Polio APS; Michael C., August 4, 1916, Box C #7, Polio APS.

104. Mrs. Elizabeth N., August 16, 1916, Box C #7, Polio APS. "I do not think this epidemic is ketching what[so]ever," Orville K., October 9, 1916, Box C #9, Polio APS.

105. T.G.S., September 11, 1916, Box C #8, Polio APS. He suggested that small springless go-carts made children vulnerable by weakening the spine.

106. E. B., August 5, 1916, Box C #3, Polio APS. Isaac R., a New York City tobacconist, warned that polio germs come from cemeteries, for when graves were dug decayed corpses were exposed, and "this fills the Air with the Infectant Germs" that spread "that Terrible Epidemic"; August 18, 1916, Box C #6, Polio APS.

107. "Skirts: The Shorter the Healthier," *Philadelphia Inquirer*, July 2, 1916.

108. Ernest J. C., July 10, 1916, Mitchel NYC.

109. Michael C., November 29, 1916, Mitchel NYC.

110. W.H.H., October 3, 1916, Box C #8, Polio APS; Kathleen D., August 29, 1916, Box C #1, Polio APS. The solution involved readjusting society's nutritional balance. Just as the Japanese had solved the problem of beriberi by giving the sick unpolished rice, so the United States could learn this lesson about nutrients and provide polio patients with "common salt." Another writer suggested additional nitrogen, "which is a Muscle Builder," by trying Clarendon Springs Waters, which, his circular noted, were "Celebrated for their Health Giving Qualities" and "Specific as a Diuretic and for Dyspepsia [&] Eczema"; G.T.M., July 11, 1916, Box C #2, Polio APS.

111. Francis F. L., July 7, 1916, Mitchel NYC. See also a letter from a Brooklyn "Committee of Citizens" with similar concerns about trash dumping; July 22, 1916, Mitchel NYC.

112. Benjamin C. M., July 7, 1916, Mitchel NYC; H.C.H., August 9, 1916, Mitchel NYC.

113. Anonymous, August 16, 1916, Box C #1, Polio APS; B.J.H., Sr., August 21, 1916, Mitchel NYC; Rosenberg, *The Cholera Years*, 121.

114. George U.A.B., August 15, 1916, Box C #7, Polio APS. On dreams to aid cancer therapy, see Patterson, *Dread Disease*, 240.

115. Mrs. L.A.L., September 2, 1916, Box C #8, Polio APS.

116. Anonymous, August 16, 1916, Box C #1, Polio APS; *New York Times*, July 29, 1916.

CHAPTER 5. A HUMBLE AND CONTRITE FRAME OF MIND

1. The mechanism of polio's transmission was not finally resolved until American researchers in the 1940s and 1950s identified the polio virus in the bloodstream and showed that it is initially an intestinal disease, usually spread by infected feces as children play with one another or through infected sewage and only rarely by water, milk, or insects; Paul, *History*, chap. 36. For an earlier version of this chapter, see Naomi Rogers, "Dirt, Flies and Immigrants: Explaining the Epidemiology of Poliomyelitis," *Journal of the History of Medicine and Allied Sciences* 44 (1989): 486–505; chapter used with permission.

2. See William Coleman, *Yellow Fever in the North: The Methods of Early Epidemiology* (Madison: University of Wisconsin Press, 1987), 173, 176–178; and see John M. Eyler, *Victorian Social Medicine: The Ideas and Methods of William Farr* (Baltimore: Johns Hopkins University Press, 1979).

3. See Franklin H. Top, ed., *The History of American Epidemiology* (St. Louis: C. V. Mosby Co., 1952); Paul, *Account of the American Epidemiological*

Society; and Abraham M. Lilienthal, ed., *Times, Places, and Persons: Aspects of the History of Epidemiology* (Baltimore: Johns Hopkins University Press, 1980).

4. See Philip D. Jordan, *The People's Health: A History of Public Health in Minnesota to 1948* (Saint Paul: Minnesota Historical Society, 1953), 91, 12, 88–89. See also "Report of the Committee of the American Medical Association on Methods for the Control of Epidemic Poliomyelitis," *Sixth Annual Report of the Commissioner of Health for the Commonwealth of Pennsylvania 1911* (Harrisburg: J.L.L. Kuhn, 1912), 76–85.

5. See *Infantile Paralysis in Massachusetts in 1909* (Boston: Wright & Potter, 1910); and *Infantile Paralysis in Massachusetts, 1907–1912.* See also Rosenkrantz, *Public Health and the State;* and Henry K. Beecher and Mark D. Altschule, *Medicine at Harvard: The First Three Hundred Years* (Hanover: University Press of New England, 1977).

6. Paul, *History,* 118–120; and Peabody, Draper and Dochez, *A Clinical Study.* Paul argued that the study's epidemiological section was written by Flexner. See also Corner, *Rockefeller Institute;* Harvey, *Science at the Bedside,* 93–95; and Saul Benison, "Speculation and Experimentation," 1–22.

7. Fee, *Disease and Discovery,* 68, 70. See also Allen Weir Freeman's autobiography, *Five Million Patients: The Professional Life of a Health Officer* (New York: Charles Scribner's Sons, 1946); Thomas B. Turner, *Heritage of Excellence: The Johns Hopkins Medical Institutions, 1914–1947* (Baltimore: Johns Hopkins University Press, 1974); and Victoria A. Harden, *Inventing the NIH: Federal Biomedical Research Policy, 1887–1937* (Baltimore: Johns Hopkins University Press, 1986).

8. See *Infantile Paralysis in Vermont, 1894–1922: A Memorial to Charles S. Caverly, M. D.* (Burlington: State Department of Public Health, 1924).

9. Paul, *History,* chap. 10; Wickman, *Acute Poliomyelitis,* 113. Wickman's study is still regarded as a classic for understanding polio's epidemiological and clinical characteristics.

10. Collins, "The Epidemiology of Poliomyelitis," 1926.

11. Wickman, *Acute Poliomyelitis,* 38. See also Paul, *History,* chap. 13. Speculating on modes of transmission Wickman noted one case of infection through a sketch and a few through milk and food, but he felt that these were rare; he also rejected theories about insects, animals, and fowls; *Acute Poliomyelitis,* 113, 118, 119.

12. For a discussion of the increased difficulty of diagnosis using the concept of abortive cases, see H. W. Hill to Simon Flexner, November 16, 1909, Polio file, Flexner papers, APS. Hill warned that because abortive cases "may or may not be poliomyelitis in fact . . . whether they are reported as such or not simply depends on the attitude of the physician concerned," 2.

13. See T. G. Hull, "A Graphical Study of Epidemiology of Poliomyelitis," *American Journal of Public Health* 7 (1917): 814.

14. Charles Bolduan, Louis C. Ager, and J. F. Terriberry, "Epidemiology of Poliomyelitis," in *Epidemic Polio: Report on the New York Epidemic of 1907 by the Collective Investigative Committee* (New York: Journal of Nervous and Mental Disease Publishing Co., no. 6, 1910), 9–27. In 1916 Haven Emerson commented that until recently polio had been regarded as a rural disease; Emerson, *Monograph*, 95.

15. Wickman, *Acute Poliomyelitis*, 38; H. W. Hill, "The Epidemiology of Anterior Poliomyelitis," *Journal of Minnesota State Medical Association and Northwestern Lancet* 29 (1909): 371.

16. See Coleman, *Yellow Fever*, chap. 1.

17. For a more detailed development of this point, see Rogers, "Germs with Legs," 599–617.

18. Rosenkrantz, *Public Health and the State*, chap. 1.

19. "Round Table," 130. See also Nicoll, "Epidemiologic Data," 234; and Freeman, "The Epidemic of Poliomyelitis in New York City, 1916," in "Studies," 108–113. The borough of Richmond had the highest precentage of children over five years (27 percent) compared to the city's overall figure of 22 percent.

20. Freeman, "Epidemic," in "Studies," 81, 84. See also Lavinder, "Richmond," in "Studies," 137–160. A study of one thousand polio cases in New York State found over half the families economically in "moderate circumstances." These investigators concluded that there was no relationship among economic status, sanitary conditions, and the appearance of the disease; Emerson, *Monograph*, 186.

21. Freeman, "Epidemic," in "Studies," 97, 133.

22. Francis E. Fronczak, "Epidemic Poliomyelitis," *New York State Journal of Medicine* 16 (1916): 390.

23. Lavinder, "Epidemic," in "Studies," 151.

24. Lavinder "Summary," in "Studies," 211–212; Frost, "Problem of Polio," in "Studies," 19, 23; Lavinder, "Richmond," in "Studies," 159. Frost concluded that the epidemic was either "nonspecific" or the result of previous exposure of unrecognized infected cases.

25. Collins, "Epidemiology of Poliomyelitis," 1928.

26. Emerson, *Monograph*, 108. Emerson noted that "anybody who goes through a hospital such as Willard Parker Hospital, with 900 children, will get an impression that these children are different physically from other children." See "Transactions," 65.

27. Freeman, "The Epidemic," in "Studies," 85.

28. Alvah H. Doty, "Special Investigation of Infantile Paralysis," manuscript, Doty file, Flexner papers, APS, 11, 15. This copy has Flexner's editorial comments throughout.

29. Rosenau, "The Mode of Transmission," 1612–1615.

30. Herbert Winslow Hill, "Discussion" during "Symposium of Epidemic Anterior Poliomyelitis" [Minnesota State Medical Association, October 12–14, 1909], *JAMA* 53 (1909): 1767. Hill found that in a 1909 Minnesota epidemic almost every case he investigated had "prolonged exposure" to dust, possibly containing infected horse feces; see Hill, "Epidemiology," 373.

31. See *Infantile Paralysis in Massachusetts;* see also Robert W. Lovett and Philip A. E. Sheppard, "The Occurrence of Infantile Paralysis in Massachusetts in 1910," *Forty-Second Annual Report of the State Board of Health of Massachusetts* (Boston: Wright & Potter, 1911), 423–435.

32. Frost, "The Problem of Polio," in "Studies," 15–16. Freeman could find no relation between low rainfall and polio and decided against Hill's dust factor; Freeman, "Epidemic," in "Studies," 81, 84.

33. Hill, "Epidemiology," 373.

34. Wade H. Frost, *Poliomyelitis (Infantile Paralysis) What Is Known of its Cause and Modes of Transmission,* Reprint no. 350 [*Public Health Reports,* July 14, 1916] (Washington, D.C.: Government Printing Office, 1916), 6, 13.

35. C. T. Brues, "Insects as Carriers of Infection: An Entomological Study of the 1916 Epidemic," in Emerson, *Monograph,* 136, 146–155. See also M. J. Rosenau and Charles T. Brues, "Some Experimental Observations upon Monkeys Concerning the Transmission of Poliomyelitis through the Agency of Stomoxys Calcitrans," *Monthly Bulletin,* Massachusetts State Board of Health (1912), reprinted in George Whipple, ed., *State Sanitation: A Review of the Work of the Massachusetts State Board of Health* (Cambridge: Harvard University Press, 1917), 358–361.

36. Mark W. Richardson, "The Rat and Infantile Paralysis—A Theory," *Transactions of the Association of American Physicians: Thirty-Third Session Held at Atlantic City, N.J., May 7 & 8, 1918,* 166. Richardson also noted the infrequency of hospital infection of doctors and nurses working with polio patients, 169. Richardson's rat theory was pursued by U.S. Public Health Service researchers studying New Jersey and Connecticut outbreaks, and some "suggestive" evidence was found, but the federal researchers rejected the theory; see Freeman, "Outside New York City," in "Studies," 190–191. Simon Flexner also asked New York City's deputy health commissioner to trap rats and mice from the "heavily infected districts" for laboratory work; Flexner to J[ohn]. S[edgwick]. Billings, July 27, 1916, Billings file, Flexner papers, APS. Billings provided over sixty rats from the Gowanas Canal area; Billings to Flexner, September 2, 1916; Flexner to Billings, September 6, 1916, Billings file, Flexner paper, APS.

37. Brues, "Insects," 158.

38. Ibid., 151, 161, 134. See also Anderson and Frost, "Transmission of Poliomyelitis," 1733–1735. For additional work on stable flies, particularly during 1913–1914, see James Warren Sever, "Anterior Poliomyelitis: A Review of the Recent Literature in Regard to the Epidemiology, Etiology, Modes

of Transmission, Bacteriology and Pathology," in *Infantile Paralysis in Massachusetts, 1907–1912*, 19–20.

39. Brues, "Insects," 137. When Henry Ling Taylor suggested that the Rockefeller Foundation fund an investigation of polio like the Thompson Commission on pellagra, perhaps he hoped for a similar insect theory conclusion; "Conference of Infantile Paralysis held at the office of [the] Rockefeller Foundation, Saturday, August 5, 1916, 10 o'clock A.M.," Flexner papers, #200/25/283, Rockefeller Archive Center, Tarrytown, New York); hereafter cited "Rockefeller Conference." See also Etheridge, *The Butterfly Caste.*

40. Henry Frauenthal and Jacolyn Van Vliet Manning, *A Manual of Infantile Paralysis with Modern Methods of Treatment Including Reports Based on the Treatment of Three Thousand Cases* (Philadelphia: F. A. Davis Co., 1914), 54.

41. Sheppard, "Acute Epidemic Poliomyelitis," 442.

42. Frost, *What Is Known*, 15. The theory of infectious secretions, he argued, was "supported by more experimental evidence" than the theory of insect transmission, 15.

43. "Rockefeller Conference," 55–56. Frost, however, commented on a few experiments with biting insects but argued that the theory had not been thoroughly confirmed; "Transactions," 66–67.

44. Herbert C. Emerson, "An Epidemic of Infantile Paralysis in Western Massachusetts in 1908," in *The Occurrence of Infantile Paralysis in Massachusetts in 1908*, ed. Lovett and Emerson (Boston: Wright & Potter, 1909), 25–26.

45. "Transactions," 81.

46. "Round Table," 142.

47. Ibid., 127–128.

48. Doty, "Special Investigation," 14.

49. Emerson, *Monograph*, 24.

50. Ibid., 23–24.

51. "Round Table," 127–128; Emerson, *Monograph*, 80. On Barren Island, see Duffy, *Public Health in New York City*, 246.

52. "Transactions," 32.

53. "Round Table," 124.

54. Ibid., 125.

55. Emerson to Flexner, January 6, 1917, Emerson file, Flexner papers, APS. Emerson hoped that "with the benefit of your advice and assistance, still further improvement on the health of the City may be accomplished."

56. Galishoff, "Great Polio Epidemic," 108. A Maine health officer told fellow officials at a Washington conference that no bottled milk was allowed in any polio sick room, only canned or breast milk; "Transactions," 141. Emerson warned mothers in New York City that, although cows could not get polio, milk could become a carrier; *New York Times,* July 7, 1916.

57. "Round Table," 131.

58. Ibid., 132.

59. Editorial, "The Infectivity of Poliomyelitis," *Medical Record*, 90 (1916): 245–246.

60. Doty, "Special Investigation," 11. See also Alvah H. Doty, *Special Investigation of Poliomyelitis 1916: Report of Committee Appointed by the Mayor to Cooperate with the Department of Health* (New York: Department of Health, 1916).

61. Doty, "Special Investigation," 11, 61, 49, 54–56.

62. Ibid., 13, 27. Freeman found only 5 percent of multiple cases in families; "The Epidemic," in "Studies," 124; Lavinder found 20 percent of multiple cases in his study of Staten Island families, although excluding "suspicious" cases the figure was only 11 percent. He could also trace 21 percent direct contact cases, but from a sample of only ninety-six cases; Lavinder, "Richmond," in "Studies," 152, 157.

63. Doty, "Special Investigation," 43, 46–47, 58. He concluded, nonetheless, that the most common means of spread were abortive cases, 57.

64. Ibid., 38–39.

65. Ibid., 58–59. He criticized the emphasis of the daily press on cleanliness for "while the value of this is obvious it does not enlighten the public concerning media of infection, *for uncleanliness and unhygienic surroundings do not generate pathogenic organisms and therefore cannot cause infectious disease*," 59.

66. "Transactions," 11–12.

67. "Round Table," 123. Newark official Charles Craster announced that the germ of polio "has yet eluded medical investigators"; *Newark Evening News*, July 6, 1916.

68. "Round Table," 134. Park noted the theory of a streptococcus as polio's infectious agent. Flexner later suggested that polio's epidemiology could best be explained by increasing viral virulence and argued that healthy carriers were rare; see Flexner, "Epidemiology of Poliomyelitis," in *Contributions to Medical and Biological Research Dedicated to Sir William Osler Bart., M.D., F. R. S. In Honour of his Seventieth Birthday July 12, 1919 by His Pupils and Co-Workers*, vol. 2 (New York: Paul B. Hoeber, 1919), 929–934; see also Louis I. Dublin, "Round Table," 126.

69. *New York Times*, August 5, 1916.

70. Lovett to Flexner, December 23, 1914; Flexner to Lovett, January 4, 1915; Lovett to Flexner, January 5, 1915; Lovett file, Flexner papers, APS.

71. Benjamin U. White with the assistance of Richard J. Wolfe and Eugene Taylor, *Stanley Cobb: A Builder of the Modern Neurosciences* (Boston: Francis C. Countway Library of Medicine, 1984), 63. I would like to thank Richard Wolfe of the Countway Medical Library at Harvard for pointing this reference out to me.

72. *New York Times*, July 26, 1916.

73. "Round Table," 129.

74. Ibid., 142.

75. "Transactions," 70.

76. Freeman, "Outside New York City," in "Studies," 191.

77. "Transactions," 114–115.

78. Ibid., 135.

79. "Round Table," 128.

EPILOGUE: POLIO SINCE FDR

1. See Finis Farr, *FDR* (New Rochelle: Arlington House, 1972), 127–128; and Hugh Gregory Gallagher, *FDR's Splendid Deception* (New York: Dodd, Mead & Co., 1988), 7; Richard Thayer Goldberg, *The Making of Franklin D. Roosevelt: Triumph Over Disability* (Cambridge: Abt Books, 1981), 26–27.

2. Farr, *FDR*, 128–130. For the theory that had he rested after the chill, the severity of the attack might have been lessened, see Gallagher, *Deception*, 1–2.

3. Goldberg, *Triumph*, 30–31.

4. Ibid., 43. Evidence of the public's and profession's continuing fear of infection and lack of a clear notion of the way polio spread reemerged when the family decided to send son James back to Groton. Lovett said it would be safe if James changed into fresh clothing and washed his hair before leaving the summer house.

5. Frank Freidel, *Franklin D. Roosevelt: The Ordeal* (Boston: Little, Brown, 1954), 121.

6. See Gallagher, *Deception*, 74, John T. Flynn, *The Roosevelt Myth* (New York: Devin Adiar, 1948), 256; Goldberg, *Triumph*, 162.

7. Farr, *FDR*, 132. Although Roosevelt himself downplayed the impact of his paralysis, a psychologist has recently argued that polio was the "central trauma" of Roosevelt's prepresidential years—a trauma that both changed him and made him president; Goldberg, *Triumph*, vii–viii.

8. Freidel, *Ordeal*, 113.

9. See Susan E. Cayleff, *Wash and Be Healed: The Water Cure Movement and Women's Health* (Philadelphia: Temple University Press, 1987).

10. Goldberg, *Triumph*, 75–76.

11. Freidel, *Ordeal*, 197. Roosevelt paid $201,667.83; Goldberg, *Triumph*, 91. By 1927 Roosevelt had closed the resort to regular guests and began fundraising to pay for its expansion and patient care; Gallagher, *Deception*, 50.

12. Freidel, *Ordeal*, 193; Turnley Walker, *Roosevelt and the Fight Against Polio* (London: Rider & Co., 1954), 80–81; Gallagher, *Deception*, 41. After regular guests complained, Roosevelt established a separate dining area and pool. For the inadequate, ineffective, and grim medical treatment available

for the disabled in the 1920s, see Gallagher, *Deception*, 28–29; Goldberg, *Triumph*, 86.

13. See Flynn, *Myth*, 256; Goldberg, *Triumph*, 110, 113; Gallagher, *Deception*, 160.

14. Jane S. Smith, *Patenting the Sun: Polio and the Salk Vaccine* (New York: William Morrow & Company, 1990), 85. For racism and segregation at Warm Springs, see Goldberg, *Triumph*, 146–151; Gallagher, *Deception*, 36; Walker, *The Fight*, 28, 35.

15. At the beginning of Roosevelt's illness, his personal advisor Louis Howe announced that it was pneumonia, before admitting polio, but he said Roosevelt had fully recovered; Gallagher, *Deception*, 18. This strategy of denial was encouraged by Roosevelt who described himself as a cured cripple or soon to be completely cured; see Gallagher, *Deception*, 78; Goldberg, *Triumph*, 131. In 1983 the wife of a former Roosevelt employee claimed that "we never, ever thought of the President as handicapped, we *never* thought of it at all"; Gallagher, *Deception*, 207. See also John Duffy, "Franklin Roosevelt: Ambiguous Symbol for Disabled Americans," *Midwest Quarterly* 29 (1987): 113–135.

16. Freidel, *Ordeal*, 251. Roosevelt's hesitancy in accepting the nomination may have also stemmed from having to accept his disability once he reentered political life; Goldberg, *Triumph*, 107. Goldberg described this period of denial lasting from 1921 to 1928; *Triumph*, 163.

17. On rumors spread by Republicans that Roosevelt suffered from spinal and brain paralysis caused by venereal disease, see Goldberg, *Triumph*, 171. On the whispering campaign that he was mentally incompetent, see Gallagher, *Deception*, 85. Georgia's governor Gene Talmadge claimed that Warm Springs was "just a racket, being disguised under the guise of charity by the President"; Gallagher, *Deception*, 147.

18. There are just three candid shots of Roosevelt: only one known picture includes his leg-braces unhidden, and only two in a wheelchair; Goldberg, *Triumph*, 127. A brief shot of Roosevelt in his wheelchair appears in the documentary film at the Roosevelt Museum at Warm Springs. The media restrictions were believed to have begun in 1928 when he told reporters, "No movies of me getting out of the machine, boys." The unspoken code was broken by *Life* magazine, which in 1937 published a photograph of Roosevelt in his wheelchair from a distance; Gallagher, *Deception*, 93–94.

19. He fell in public at least three times, including at the Philadelphia Democratic convention in 1936, but his falls were not reported by the press; Gallagher, *Deception*, 101. On the tricks used by Roosevelt to maintain this image, including his naval cape, his fedora, and his cigarette holder, see Gallagher, *Deception*, 213. Gallagher noted that most biographers have treated polio as simply an episode in Roosevelt's prepresidential career, but this approach reflects the way Roosevelt presented himself and ignores the extraordinary cost in energy used to maintain this image; *Deception*, 210.

20. Goldberg, *Triumph*, 205, 164; Paul, *History*, 304.

21. Aaron E. Klein, *Trial By Fury: The Polio Vaccine Controversy* (New York: Charles Scribner's Sons, 1972), 15–16. They became known as "Paralysis Dances"; Paul, *History*, 305. The Foundation's decision to fund polio patients without a means test drew some criticism; Smith, *Patenting the Sun*, 69–70.

22. Cantor was probably alluding to a contemporary newsreel documentary, "The March of Times"; Klein, *Fury*, 17; Roland H. Berg, *Polio and Its Problems* (Philadelphia: J. B. Lippincott, 1948), 60–61.

23. Paul de Kruif, *The Fight for Life* (New York: Harcourt, Brace & Co., 1938), 145.

24. Richard Carter, *Breakthrough: The Saga of Jonas Salk* (New York: Trident Press, 1962), 84.

25. Smith, *Patenting the Sun*, 319, 83.

26. Paul de Kruif, *The Sweeping Wind: A Memoir* (New York: Harcourt, Brace & World, 1962), 177.

27. De Kruif was "the sort of science advisor you picked if you knew very little about the business of research"; Smith, *Patenting the Sun*, 71.

28. De Kruif knew about "the glamour of medical research" and how to turn it on; Paul, *History*, 305.

29. De Kruif, *Sweeping Wind*, 179, 178; de Kruif, *Fight for Life*, 169–170; Smith, *Patenting the Sun*, 72. There were at least twelve cases of polio and six deaths. Brodie's vaccine was based on the virus in monkeys' spinal cords and weakened the virus by formalin, a solution of formaldehyde. Brodie died four years later, possibly a suicide; Smith, *Patenting the Sun*, 132.

30. Paul described it as "brief setback"; *History*, 304. He noted that the committee also gave grants to researchers at Johns Hopkins, University of Pennsylvania, Harvard, and Yale; *History*, 306.

31. De Kruif, *Sweeping Wind*, 201–202. Thomas D. Spies, of Birmingham, Alabama, had developed theories about the role of nutrition in polio after his successful work on the role of niacin in preventing pellagra. De Kruif resigned in 1941.

32. Paul, *History*, 304. The Foundation, a "very large, very slick organization," used "just about any gimmick"; Smith, *Patenting the Sun*, 84, 80.

33. It drew the public's consciousness "to a degree close to hysteria"; Paul, *History*, 310–312; Gallagher, *Deception*, 157. Paul argued that the Foundation used only 11 percent of its full budget for research grants compared to 13 percent for fund-raising; *History*, 312.

34. Ibid., 309. Paul argued that scientists associated Madison Avenue with "pseudo-science."

35. Ibid., 311. Established scientists saw the Foundation as a "gift horse"; ibid., 316; and see Smith, *Patenting the Sun*, 98.

36. Paul, *History*, 318. For an opposing view, see Benison, "The History of Polio Research," 308–343.

37. See de Kruif, *Fight for Life*, 154.

38. Not until the 1940s did the new electron microscope provide researchers with a clear picture of the polio virus. Penicillin and streptomycin eliminated contaminating bacteria and allowed scientists to use human intestine tissue.

39. In 1935, at Flexner's suggestion, Rockefeller scientists Albert Sabin and Peter Olitsky had tested the intestinal theory on human embryo tissue. Using Flexner's MV virus they had shown that the virus would grow only on nerve tissue; Greer Williams, *Virus Hunters* (New York: Alfred A. Knopf, 1960), 249. It was "one of those unfortunate accidents of science" that they had used this neurotropic strain; Klein, *Fury*, 58. Paul agreed that "the choice of the MV strain was unfortunate"; *History*, 373; and see Carter, *Breakthrough*, 90–91.

40. Paul, *History*, 374–381.

41. Ibid., 346–352. In 1916, 95 percent of reported polio cases were birth to nine years; in 1940, 65 percent were under ten years, and 24 percent were ten to nineteen years; and in 1947, 52 percent were birth to nine, and 38 percent were ten to nineteen. On the appearance of polio narratives written by adult victims in the 1940s and 1950s, see Daniel J. Wilson, "Covenants of Work and Grace: Themes of Recovery and Redemption in Polio Narratives" (Paper presented at American Association for the History of Medicine, annual meeting, Cleveland, Ohio, 1991).

42. Paul, *History*, 360–363. In 1946 Paul found almost 100 percent polio antibodies in North African children and strikingly low levels in American children. This suggested that polio was a "worldwide endemic infection of infancy" and introduced him to the new science of serological epidemiology; Paul, *History*, 364, 367. On work by both Isabel Morgan and William Hammon, which showed that serum antibodies could protect polio-infected monkeys, see Paul, *History*, 385, 387.

43. Ibid., 382–383, 387.

44. Ibid., 387. The theory argued that if the virus went directly to the central nervous system, then it was not accessible to the action of the body's natural defences such as circulating antibodies; ibid., 383–384. See also de Kruif, *Fight for Life*, 171; Berg, *Problems*, 71; Dorothy M. Horstmann, "The Poliomyelitis Story: A Scientific Hegira," *Yale Journal of Biology and Medicine* 58 (1985): 82.

45. Paul, *History*, 385.

46. Charles Armstrong, a Public Health Service researcher, and Edwin Schultz, a bacteriologist at Stanford University, developed chemical nasal sprays using picric acid and zinc sulfate, which were tested in trials in Ala-

bama and North Carolina in 1936 and Toronto and Chicago in 1937; Paul, *History*, 272; Berg, *Problems*, 34–47. Schultz received funding from the Birthday Ball Commission for his experiments, which were based on the theory of a natural protein in the mucous membrane that could form a protective coating around the nerve ending; Berg, *Problems*, 37. The results of the Toronto trials showed only a 1 percent difference; Berg, *Problems*, 40–43. See also de Kruif, *Fight for Life*, 187–193; and Naomi Rogers, "Trial and Error: Polio Prevention and Public Health in Alabama in 1936" (Paper presented at Organization of American Historians, annual meeting, Louisville, Kentucky, 1991).

47. Williams, *Virus Hunters*, 267; see also Carter, *Breakthrough*, 86–87; Horstmann, "Scientific Hegira," 83.

48. Paul, *History*, 375; and see Williams, *Virus Hunters*, 252–255.

49. Smith also repeated the "left over theory"; *Patenting the Sun*, 126; and on Enders and his team as the "three princes of Serendip," see Williams, *Virus Hunters*, 251. But Paul presented Enders's discovery not as an accident but as part of a carefully controlled study and agreed that it "changed the course of polio research"; *History*, 375–376. For a suggestion that Enders tested the polio virus because he was funded by the Foundation that had given his laboratory "abundant" polio sources, see Allan Chase, *Magic Shots: A Human and Scientific Account of the Long and Continuing Struggle to Eradicate Infectious Diseases by Vaccination* (New York: William Morrow & Co., 1982), 291.

50. The Foundation began this funding in the late 1930s and also developed respiratory centers and training programs for therapists, Paul, *History*, 331–333. The iron lung raised difficult ethical questions over whether patients should stay there the rest of their lives and, when respirators were limited, who should be chosen; Paul, *History*, 330.

51. English physicians had first introduced strict casts and splinting after rejecting active physical therapy, a policy then adopted by American therapists; Berg, *Problems*, 124–125. This policy was taken "to excess"; Paul, *History*, 338–340. On conflicting assessments of Kenny, see Berg, *Problems*, 132–147; and Victor Cohn, *Sister Kenny: The Woman Who Challenged the Doctors* (Minneapolis: University of Minnesota Press, 1975).

52. Many physicians today have rejected Kenny's hot pack theory but have continued her stress on exercising paralyzed muscles; Dowling, *Fighting Infection*, 207. On the "raging controversy" between Kenny and the medical profession, see Berg, *Problems*, 125–133. Paul argued that health professionals needed a "vigorous personality" to attack the splinting regime and noted the popular belief that there was something magical in Kenny herself as well as her methods; Paul, *History*, 340–345.

53. Klein, *Fury*, 46; the conferences were intended "to enliven the tempo of polio research without seeming to prod"; Carter, *Breakthrough*, 108; and see Paul, *History*, 320–322.

54. See Berg, *Problems*, 63–77, 108–110. On the Foundation's hope that "the door to chemotherapy is ajar; the pill for polio may yet be found," see Berg, *Problems*, 77.

55. On the "sharp differences" on immunization methods, see Paul, *History*, 401; Smith, *Patenting the Sun*, 146–149.

56. Paul, *History*, 400–402; Smith, *Patenting the Sun*, 109–110, 124. The Hopkins researchers were David Bodian, Howard Howe, and Isabel Morgan; those from Yale were John Paul, James Trask, and Dorothy Horstmann.

57. Dowling, *Fighting Infection*, 211.

58. See Carter, *Breakthrough*, 41–42; Smith, *Patenting the Sun*, 147–148.

59. Smith, *Patenting the Sun*, 103–106; Paul, *History*, 430–431.

60. Smith, *Patenting the Sun*, 137–139. "Fortunately the trials came out all right"; Paul, *History*, 417–418. Either Salk did not mention his test on retarded children to the Foundation (Carter, *Breakthrough*, 100), or he was coached by Weaver to phrase his work tactfully (Smith, *Patenting the Sun*, 138–139).

61. Paul, *History*, 422; Williams, *Virus Hunters*, 231–233; and see Allan M. Brandt, "Polio, Politics, Publicity, and Duplicity: Ethical Aspects in the Development of the Salk Vaccine," *International Journal of Health Sciences* 8 (1978): 257–270. Thomas Francis, Jr., insisted on equal numbers of placebos and no interference from the Foundation. The trials used two groups of controls: injected (placebos) and observed; Paul, *History*, 427. Altogether 1,829,916 children in 211 areas of forty-four states participated; Paul, *History*, 427 n.3.

62. On behalf of the Foundation O'Connor bought up all American supplies of gamma globulin and agreed to let federal health officials distribute it; Carter, *Breakthrough*, 104–105. Gamma globulin had been used to fight measles and viral hepatitis during the Korean War, but the Foundation, unenthusiastic about its use against polio, feared that the trauma from the injection could cause vulnerability to polio and the public would dislike control groups; Paul, *History*, 392–394. But the trials were organized and promoted by William Hammon who became a popular hero; Klein, *Fury*, 60–62, 70. Paul argued that scientists had established evidence of the polio virus in blood *before* the revival of interest in preventive serum; Paul, *History*, 389–390. But Carter argued that *after* the gamma globulin trials Bodian and Horstmann looked for the virus in the blood and found it; *Breakthrough*, 132.

63. "The foundation had brought the public pressure on itself"; Klein, *Fury*, 94.

64. Smith, *Patenting the Sun*, 288. The field trials cost $7 million.

65. Williams, *Virus Hunters*, 313.

66. Paul, *History*, 405.

67. Maurice Brodie had been assistant professor at New York University. Salk later developed a killed-virus vaccine using formaldehyde, as Brodie

had; Klein, *Fury*, 85. On a positive comparison between Salk and Edward Jenner, see Williams, *Virus Hunters*, 354–355.

68. Paul, *History*, 423–424, 443–444; Klein, *Fury*, 81–84. The trial meeting "had many features of a Hollywood extravaganza—features that were far from pleasing to the scientific community"; Horstmann, "Scientific Hegira," 85. The vaccine had an immediate impact in the United States: in 1954 there were 13.9 cases per 100,000; in 1961, 0.5.

69. Smith, *Patenting the Sun*, 364–367. The vaccine was the suspected cause because a number of victims developed paralysis in their left arms. Salk cooperated with the families that later sued the Cutter laboratory. The courts compensated families but did not find that Cutter had knowingly produced a faulty product; Smith, *Patenting the Sun*, 367.

70. After investigators found nothing unusual at the Cutter laboratories, many began to attack Salk's methods of inactivation and his use of the strong Mahoney strain. Later it was discovered that in mass production the vaccine required extra filtration to make sure that the virus did not "clump" together making it difficult to be affected by formalin; Smith, *Patenting the Sun*, 363–366; Williams, *Virus Hunters*, 336–340. Carter, however, claimed that the vaccine was prepared "in violation or ignorance" of Salk's theories; *Breakthrough*, 125.

71. See Klein, *Fury*, 59, 130–131; Carter, *Breakthrough*, 97. They fed live virus to the children in chocolate milk, and found twenty children developed polio antibodies; Carter, *Breakthrough*, 109–111.

72. Klein, *Fury*, 135–136, 140–141; Paul, *History*, 452. The ethical problems concern the use of human subjects for medical trials; the Articles of Nuremberg on the legal capacity to give consent were not followed in polio trials; Paul, *History*, 408. Salk often said later that it would be impossible to repeat his polio work with recent human-subject review boards; Smith, *Patenting the Sun*, 137–139.

73. Carter, *Breakthrough*, 81–82, 90, 111–117. Carter described their relations as "open warfare."

74. Klein, *Fury*, 138; Paul, *History*, 445; Chase, *Magic Shots*, 281. Paul described Sabin as not only an "able, tireless, and articulate medical scientist" but also as egotistic and possessive; *History*, 445.

75. Sabin had already had experience with a live-virus vaccine through his work on dengue fever and encephalitis during World War II; Paul, *History*, 448.

76. Klein, *Fury*, 140–141. It was "probably not wise" for the Foundation to have discouraged a live-virus vaccine; Paul, *History*, 420.

77. Paul, *History*, 455–459.

78. These communities had not wanted a "Soviet-tested" vaccine; Klein, *Fury,* 142–143, 145–177; Paul, *History,* 462–464.

79. Klein, *Fury,* 146.

80. Ibid., 147.

81. Alistair MacLean, *The Satan Bug* (Greenwich: Fawcett, 1962), 42.

82. Paul, *History,* 465–467. For Type I, the risk was one or less in a million, Type II had no measurable risk, and Type III was restricted to those under eighteen; Dowling, *Fighting Infection,* 218.

83. Klein, *Fury,* 154; see also Williams, *Virus Hunters,* 351.

84. Klein, *Fury,* 157, 9.

85. Paul, *History,* 404, 405.

86. Ibid., 433; Elizabeth Etheridge, "The CDC Establishes Its Credibility" (manuscript, 1989), 20.

87. De Kruif, *Fight for Life,* 157. For a similar critique, see Benison, "History of Polio Research," 308–310.

88. Smith, *Patenting the Sun,* 98–99.

89. Carter, *Breakthrough,* 87, 88.

90. Smith, *Patenting the Sun,* 367. The response to the Cutter incident was "predictable and unedifying. Without exception, everyone blamed somebody else"; *Patenting the Sun,* 360.

91. Dowling, *Fighting Infection,* 218, 219. Dowling also noted "the unwillingness to leave the final decisions on research support in the hands of the experts."

92. Smith, *Patenting the Sun,* 184. Enders was said to have called Salk's work "quackery"; Carter, *Breakthrough,* 88.

93. Smith, *Patenting the Sun,* 207; and see Carter, *Breakthrough,* 107–108.

94. See Carter, *Breakthrough,* 299–300; Smith, *Patenting the Sun,* 336–337.

95. Smith, *Patenting the Sun,* 374–377. Smith noted that his stature as a popular hero has risen over the years as his real influence has waned; *Patenting the Sun,* 387.

96. Paul, *History,* 440, 451; Dowling, *Fighting Infection,* 218. In *Breakthrough* Carter strongly argued in favor of the Salk vaccine. For the continuing debate between Salk and Sabin, see *New York Times,* February 4, 1988.

97. Horstmann, "Scientific Hegira," 88; Klein, *Fury,* 149–150. "It is a rare biological product with a high degree of effectiveness that exhibits complete safety"; Paul, *History,* 467.

98. Paul, *History,* 429, 432, 415.

99. During the 1955 congressional hearings John Paul criticized the popular belief that science was a "fixed thing"; Klein, *Fury,* 120–121.

100. Paul, *History,* 467.

101. Smith, *Patenting the Sun*, 77, 238. We have little idea of the life, career choices, and work of polio scientists Dorothy Horstmann and Isabel Morgan. Even Elizabeth Kenny lacks a full scholarly biography.

102. See Goldberg, *Triumph*, 37, 67, 73; Gallagher, *Deception*, 80; Freidel, *Ordeal*, 119.

103. It employed former patients as officials, staff, and teachers; Gallagher, *Deception*, 55.

104. Ibid., 63, 95. Gallagher noted that after Roosevelt's death all the ramps to Roosevelt's Little White House were removed, and the place was not accessible to the physically disabled until the Bartlett Act of 1968; ibid., 208–209.

105. See Klein, *Fury*, for the title of his first chapter.

106. Berg, *Problems*, 156; and see Williams, *Virus Hunters*, 241.

107. Klein, *Fury*, 151. Supposedly Salk's first words were "dirt, dirt"; Carter, *Breakthrough*, 29.

108. Smith, *Patenting the Sun*, 72–73.

109. See U. Alsentzer, "Post-polio Syndrome," *North Carolina Medical Journal* 47 (1986): 399–400; E. W. Streib, "Post-polio Syndrome: A Common Condition in Need of Recognition," *Iowa Medicine* 79 (1989): 115–119.

110. Emerson, *Monograph*, 298.

Bibliographic Essay

In the 1980s there has been an increasing interest in the history of twentieth-century medicine and disease. In part, this has been a reaction to the attacks on medical authority and expertise during the 1960s and 1970s. In reassessing the influence of science on society and the professionalization of physicians on health care, historians have become both more critical of medical science and more conscious of its powers. A new interest in social and cultural history has focused attention on the words and actions of ordinary physicians, health officials, and patients and urged a multidimensional approach to medical history.

MEDICAL RESEARCH AND PRACTICE
For some helpful analyses of the cultural authority of science and its influence on health policy and the medical profession, see Rosemary Stevens, *American Medicine and the Public Interest* (New Haven: Yale University Press, 1970); George Rosen, *The Structure of American Medical Practice, 1875–1941*, ed. Charles E. Rosenberg (1976; reprint, Philadelphia: University of Pennsylvania Press, 1983); Russell C. Maulitz, " 'Physician versus Bacteriologist': The Ideology of Science in Clinical Medicine," in *The Therapeutic Revolution: Essays in the Social History of American Medicine*, ed. Morris J. Vogel and Charles E. Rosenberg (Philadelphia: University of Pennsylvania Press, 1979), 99–108; Paul Starr, *The Social Transformation of American Medicine* (New York: Basic Books, 1982); and Barbara Gutmann Rosenkrantz, "The Search

for Professional Order in 19th-Century American Medicine," in *Sickness and Health in America: Readings in the History of Medicine and Public Health,* ed. Judith Walzer Leavitt and Ronald L. Numbers (Madison: University of Wisconsin Press, 1985), 219–232.

Scientists and clinicians worked in and shaped specific institutions. I found George Corner's study helpful if at times evangelical: George W. Corner, *A History of the Rockefeller Institute, 1901–1953: Origins and Growth* (New York: Rockefeller Institute Press, 1964); and see Isabel R. Plesset, *Noguchi and His Patrons* (Rutherford: Farleigh Dickinson University Press, 1980). Useful for the broader social context of relations between philanthropy and science research is E. Richard Brown, *Rockefeller Medicine Men: Medicine and Capitalism in America* (Berkeley: University of California Press, 1979). On popular critiques of the new sciences and the response of scientists, see Susan Eyrich Lederer, "Hideyo Noguchi's Luetin Experiment and the Antivivisectionists," *Isis* 76 (1985): 31–48; and Lederer, "Human Experimentation and Antivivisection in Turn-of-the-Century America" (Ph.D. diss., University of Wisconsin-Madison, 1987). For a discussion of aspects of the history of the United States Public Health Service, see Ralph C. Williams, *The United States Public Health Service, 1798–1950* (Washington, D.C.: Commissioned Officers Association, 1951); Victoria A. Harden, *Inventing the NIH: Federal Biomedical Research Policy, 1887–1937* (Baltimore: Johns Hopkins University Press, 1986); and Elizabeth Etheridge's study of the Centers for Disease Control (CDC) (University of California Press, forthcoming).

Medical historians have only recently begun to pay attention to the practice of physicians, and the routine work of twentieth-century physicians and clinical specialists is still largely unexplored. For an understanding of the broader intellectual tradition of medical practice I have relied on two important works about nineteenth-century therapeutics: Charles E. Rosenberg, "The Therapeutic Revolution: Medicine, Meaning and Social Change in Nineteenth-Century America," in *The Therapeutic Revolution: Essays in the Social History of American Medicine,* ed. Morris J. Vogel and Charles E. Rosenberg (Philadelphia: University of Pennsylvania Press, 1979), 3–25; and John Harley Warner, *The Therapeutic Perspective: Medical Practice, Knowledge, and Identity in America, 1820–1885* (Cambridge: Harvard University Press, 1986). For a brief overview of twentieth-century therapies, see Harry F. Dowling, *Fighting Infection: Conquests of the Twentieth Century* (Cambridge: Harvard University Press, 1977).

PUBLIC HEALTH

In the past two decades medical and social historians have made pub
lic health history a lively field. They have sought to integrate public
health theory and practice and examined the new laboratory sciences
within the context of civic reform. For a useful overview of public
health and its place in American medicine, see George Rosen, *A History of Public Health* (New York: MD Publications, 1958). On public
health and social reform, see Richard A. Meckel, *Save the Babies: American Public Health Reform and the Prevention of Infant Mortality, 1850–
1929* (Baltimore: Johns Hopkins University Press, 1990).

For insightful reflections on the filth theory of disease and sanitary
science, see Lloyd G. Stevenson, "Science Down the Drain: On the
Hostility of Certain Sanitarians to Animal Experimentation, Bacteriology, and Immunology," *Bulletin of the History of Medicine* 29 (1955): 1–26;
James H. Cassedy, "The Flamboyant Colonel Waring: An Anticontagionist Holds the American Stage in the Age of Pasteur and
Koch," *Bulletin of the History of Medicine* 36 (1962): 163–176; and especially Charles E. Rosenberg, "Florence Nightingale on Contagion: The
Hospital as Moral Universe," in *Healing and History: Essays for George
Rosen*, ed. Rosenberg (New York: Science History Publications, 1979),
116–136. An important case study of nineteenth-century urban public
health is Judith Walzer Leavitt, *The Healthiest City: Milwaukee and the
Politics of Health Reform* (Princeton: Princeton University Press, 1982),
see also Philip D. Jordan, *The People's Health: A History of Public Health
in Minnesota to 1948* (Saint Paul: Minnesota Historical Society, 1953);
and Stuart Galishoff, *Safeguarding the Public Health: Newark, 1895–
1918* (Westport: Greenwood Press, 1975). The post-1890 medical history of New York City and State has had many chroniclers; for two
important scholarly accounts, see John Duffy, *A History of Public Health
in New York City, 1866–1966*, vol. 2 (New York: Russell Sage Foundation, 1974); and David A. Blancher, " 'Workshops of the Bacteriological Revolution': A History of the Laboratories of the New York City
Department of Health, 1892–1912" (Ph.D. diss., City University of
New York, 1979). For Philadelphia, see Edward T. Morman, "Clinical
Pathology in America, 1865–1915: Philadelphia as a Test Case," *Bulletin of the History of Medicine* 58 (1984): 198–214; and Morman, "Scientific Medicine Comes to Philadelphia: Public Health Transformed,
1854–1899" (Ph.D. diss., University of Pennsylvania, 1986).

An imporant study of the transformation of American public health
from sanitary science to the New Public Health is Barbara Gutmann

Rosenkrantz, *Public Health and the State: Changing Views in Massachusetts, 1842–1936* (Cambridge: Harvard University Press, 1972). See also Elizabeth Fee, *Disease and Discovery: A History of the Johns Hopkins School of Public Health and Hygiene, 1916–1939* (Baltimore: Johns Hopkins University Press, 1987); and Barbara Gutmann Rosenkrantz, "Cart Before Horse: Theory, Practice and Professional Image in American Public Health, 1870–1920," *Journal of the History of Medicine* 29 (1974): 55–73. The New Public Health movement demands further scholarly investigation, but an important starting point is James H. Cassedy, *Charles V. Chapin and the Public Health Movement* (Cambridge: Harvard University Press, 1962). For recent brief studies of public health in its social and urban context, see Daniel M. Fox, "Social Policy and City Politics: Tuberculosis Reporting in New York, 1889–1900," *Bulletin of the History of Medicine* 49 (1975): 169–175; Suellen M. Hoy, " 'Municipal Housekeeping': The Role of Women in Improving Urban Sanitation Practices, 1880–1917," in *Pollution and Reform in American Cities, 1870–1930,* ed. Martin V. Melosi (Austin: University of Texas Press, 1980), 173–198; and Charles E. Rosenberg, "Making It in Urban Medicine: A Career in the Age of Scientific Medicine," *Bulletin of the History of Medicine* 64 (1990): 163–186. On the germ theory of disease, see Phyllis A. Richmond, "The Germ Theory of Disease," in *Times, Places and Persons: Aspects of the History of Epidemiology,* ed. Abraham M. Lilienthal (Baltimore: Johns Hopkins University Press, 1980); Andrew McClary, "Germs Are Everywhere: The Germ Threat as Seen in Magazine Articles, 1890–1920," *Journal of American Culture* 3 (1980): 32–46; Naomi Rogers, "Germs with Legs: Flies, Disease and the New Public Health," *Bulletin of the History of Medicine* 63 (1989): 599–617; and Nancy Tomes, "The Private Side of Public Health: Sanitary Science, Domestic Hygiene, and the Germ Theory, 1870–1900," *Bulletin of the History of Medicine* 64 (1990): 509–539.

DISEASE

My starting point for this study was, as it is for many medical historians, Charles E. Rosenberg, *The Cholera Years: The United States in 1832, 1849, and 1866* (Chicago: University of Chicago Press, 1962). Spurred partly by the AIDS epidemic and also by an increasing interest in disease as a window to social and cultural tensions, the 1970s and 1980s have seen a series of histories exploring twentieth-century diseases. Most of this work focuses on disease as a public health problem, but much of it also examines the political, economic, social, and moral issues raised by professional and popular responses to disease.

Of the works on tuberculosis I found useful René Dubos and Jean Dubos, *The White Plague: Tuberculosis, Man and Society* (1952; reprint, New Brunswick: Rutgers University Press, 1987); Michael E. Teller, *The Tuberculosis Movement: A Public Health Campaign in the Progressive Era* (Westport: Greenwood Press, 1988); and Georgiana Danielle Feldberg, " 'An Antitoxin of Self Respect': North American Debates over Vaccination against Tuberculosis, 1890–1960" (Ph.D. diss., Harvard University, 1989). For disease and health policy, see Elizabeth W. Etheridge, *The Butterfly Caste: A Social History of Pellagra in the South* (Westport: Greenwood Press, 1972); Alfred W. Crosby, *America's Forgotten Pandemic: The Influenza of 1918* (1978; reprint, Cambridge: Cambridge University Press, 1989); Allan M. Brandt, *No Magic Bullet: A Social History of Venereal Disease in the United States from 1880* (New York: Oxford University Press, 1985); James T. Patterson, *The Dread Disease: Cancer and Modern American Culture* (Cambridge: Harvard University Press, 1987); and Victoria A. Harden, *Rocky Mountain Spotted Fever: History of a Twentieth-Century Disease* (Baltimore: Johns Hopkins University Press, 1990). For philanthropy and public health, see John Ettling, *The Germ of Laziness: Rockefeller Philanthropy and Public Health in the New South* (Cambridge; Harvard University Press, 1981). For disease history presented explicitly within an AIDS framework, see Elizabeth Fee and Daniel M. Fox, eds., *AIDS: The Burdens of History* (Berkeley: University of California Press, 1988).

Polio

Polio records have been surprisingly neglected by historians, perhaps a result of a sense that by the 1960s scientists had truly conquered the disease and left little to be discussed. For my study of polio between 1900 and 1920 I sampled local English-language newspapers: *New York Times, Newark Evening News, Philadelphia Inquirer,* and *Philadelphia Evening Bulletin.* Other studies using immigrant language sources need to be explored. I also read the *Annual Reports* of state health boards in New York, New Jersey, Pennsylvania, and Massachusetts, the reports by New York City and Philadelphia health departments, and the minutes of state and local departments. I found most of these sources more helpful for a broad public health context than for specific discussions of efforts to combat polio. More useful were special investigations undertaken by municipal, state, and Rockefeller Institute investigators: see *Epidemic Polio: Report on the New York Epidemic of 1907 by the Collective Investigative Committee* (New York: Journal of Nervous and Mental Disease Publishing Co., no. 6, 1910); Francis C.

Peabody, George Draper, and A. R. Dochez, *A Clinical Study of Acute Poliomyelitis* (New York: Rockefeller Institute of Medical Research, no. 4, June 1, 1912); C. H. Lavinder, A. W. Freeman, and W. H. Frost, "Epidemiological Studies of Poliomyelitis in New York City and the North-Eastern United States during the Year 1916," *Public Health Bulletin* 91 (1918); "Transactions of a Special Conference of State and Territorial Health Officers with the United States Public Health Service, for the Consideration of the Prevention of the Spread of Poliomyelitis: Held at Washington, D.C., August 17 and 18, 1916," *Public Health Bulletin* 83 (1917); and especially Haven Emerson, *A Monograph on The Epidemic of Poliomyelitis (Infantile Paralysis) in New York City in 1916. Based on the Official Reports of the Bureaus of the Department of Health* (New York: Department of Health, 1917).

For responses by physicians and clinical investigators I relied on articles in *Journal of the American Medical Association,* in local medical journals such as *New York State Medical Journal, New York Medical Journal, American Medicine* and *Medical Record,* and in specialist journals such as *American Journal of Diseases of Children* and *Archives of Pediatrics.* Useful for the European context were Ivar Wickman, *Acute Poliomyelitis (Heine-Medin's Disease),* translated by J.W.A.W. Maloney (1907; New York: Journal of Nervous and Mental Disease, no. 16, 1913), and Paul H. Roemer, *Epidemic Infantile Paralysis (Heine-Medin Disease),* translated by H. Ridley Prentice (1911; London: John Bale, Sons & Daniellson, 1913). Epidemiological studies of polio were published in numerous journals and collections, but see, in particular, *Infantile Paralysis in Vermont, 1894–1922: A Memorial to Charles S. Caverly, M.D.* (Burlington: State Department of Public Health, 1924); *Infantile Paralysis in Massachusetts, 1907–1912* (Boston: Wright and Potter, 1914); and Kenneth F. Maxcy, ed., *Papers of Wade Hampton Frost: A Contribution to Epidemiological Method* (New York: Commonwealth Fund, 1941). My interest in this topic made me aware of the lack of historical interest in American epidemiology. For brief introductions, see Franklin H. Top, ed., *The History of American Epidemiology* (St. Louis: C. V. Mosby Co., 1952); and John R. Paul, *An Account of the American Epidemiological Society: A Retrospect of Some Fifty Years* (New Haven: Yale Journal of Biology and Medicine: Academic Press, 1973); and Abraham M. Lilienthal, ed. *Times, Places and Persons: Aspects of the History of Epidemiology* (Baltimore: Johns Hopkins University Press, 1980). For a recent study that presents epidemiological practice as an integral part of social and intellectual history, see William Coleman, *Yellow Fever in the North: The*

Methods of Early Epidemiology (Madison: University of Wisconsin Press, 1987).

Historians of twentieth-century medicine who wish to study public perceptions of disease know well the difficulties of finding diaries and letters, for until recently many archivists tended to think that any post-1900 document was "not old enough to save." For comments on the lay perspective, I have relied partly on memoirs and biographies of figures who helped to shape polio health policy: Allen Weir Freeman, *Five Million Patients: The Professional Life of a Health Officer* (New York: Charles Scribner's Sons, 1946); and Charles-Edward Amory Winslow, *The Life of Hermann M. Biggs: Physician and Statesman of the Public Health* (Philadelphia: Lea & Febiger, 1929). I was lucky enough to find two caches of letters by lay men and women, one in the New York City Municipal Archives and the other in Simon Flexner's papers at the American Philosophical Society in Philadelphia, as well as occasional letters in newspapers and at the National Archives in Washington, D.C. I am very grateful that medical historian James Harvey Young gave me copies of letters his father, a pastor in New York City, wrote to his mother during the 1916 epidemic.

Most histories of polio written over the past thirty years have been written by protagonists. For the most useful, see John R. Paul, *A History of Poliomyelitis* (New Haven: Yale University Press, 1971); Paul F. Clark, "History of Poliomyelitis Up to the Present Time," in *Infantile Paralysis: A Symposium Delivered at Vanderbilt University April, 1941* (New York: National Foundation for Infantile Paralysis, 1941), 3–33; and Dorothy M. Horstmann "The Poliomyelitis Story: A Scientific Hegira," *Yale Journal of Biology and Medicine* 58 (1985): 79–90. The most important senior scholar of polio history is Saul Benison, who has published a series of studies of polio research. See Saul Benison, "The History of Polio Research in the United States: Appraisal and Lessons," in *The Twentieth Century Sciences: Studies in the Biography of Ideas*, ed. Gerald Holton (New York: W. W. Norton, 1972), 308–343; Benison, "Poliomyelitis and the Rockefeller Institute: Social Effects and Institutional Response," *Journal of the History of Medicine* 29 (1974): 74–93; and Benison, "Speculation and Experimentation in Early Poliomyelitis Research," *Clio Medica* 10 (1975): 1–22. An unusual and insightful study is Benison's annotated oral history of polio virologist Thomas Rivers. This work contains reflections on aspects of polio research from the 1910s to the 1960s with tantalizing comments by both Rivers and Benison; Benison, ed., *Tom Rivers: Reflections on a Life in Medicine and Science* (Cambridge: MIT Press, 1967). For other aspects of polio history, see Stuart Galishoff, "Newark and the Great Polio Epidemic of 1916," *New Jersey History* 54 (1976): 101–111; and Allan M. Brandt, "Polio, Politics, Publicity, and Duplicity: Ethical Aspects in the Development of the Salk Vaccine," *International Journal of the Health Sciences* 8 (1978): 257–270.

There is still no full history of the National Foundation for Infantile Paralysis, but other issues in polio history have recently received attention. See Jane S. Smith, *Patenting the Sun: Polio and the Salk Vaccine* (New York: William Morrow & Co., 1990), and Richard Thayer Goldberg, *The Making of Franklin D. Roosevelt: Triumph Over Disability* (Cambridge: Abt Books, 1981). For a discussion of these and additional works in greater depth I refer the reader to the Epilogue.

Index

Abramson, Harry L., 83–84, 94
Acquired Immune Deficiency Syndrome (AIDS), 3, 6–7, 166, 189
American Cancer Society, 172
American Cynamid Company, 180
American Epidemiological Society, 27, 140
American Heart Association, 172
American Journal of Diseases of Children, 83
American Journal of Electrotherapeutics and Radiology, 93
American Journal of Public Health, 56
American Museum of Natural History (New York City), 9, 14, 21
American Public Health Association, 140
Anderson, John F., 62, 81, 95
animals: as disease carriers, 42, 59, 117, 126, 139, 145, 150–152, 156, 161, 207n122; as laboratory subjects, 22–24, 58, 77–78, 81–82, 89, 99, 103, 106, 117, 138, 151, 173, 204n99; cats, 10, 58, 68, 205n103; chickens, 82, 135; cows, 124, 127; dogs, 58, 60, 68; frogs, 117; guinea pigs, 82–83; horses, 68, 99, 117, 150–151, 158; mice, 126, 173; rabbits, 58, 82; rats, 152, 173. *See also* monkeys

antibiotics, 24, 173
anti-polio serum, *see* serum
anti-Semitism, 177, 185. *See also* immigrants
antitoxins, 17, 73; diphtheria, 17, 87, 89, 96, 102, 117, 122; tetanus, 96
anti-vaccination movement, 102, 116
antivivisectionists, 22, 185
Apple, Rima, 108
Armstrong, Charles, 173
Asbury Park Baby Parade, 43

bacteria, *see* germs
bacteriologists, 36, 172
bacteriology, 4, 16–19, 31, 70, 73–74, 104, 110, 122–124, 144, 163; model of polio, 82, 138, 162
Barbour, Philip F., 90–91
Barren Island (New York), 156
Behring, Emil, 28, 96, 103
Benison, Saul, 23
Biggs, Hermann, 26, 36, 59, 62
blacks, 13, 142, 156. *See also* race
blood: for diagnosis, 74, 78, 178; for polio diagnosis, 76, 79, 85, 87, 116–117; and polio pathology, 23–24, 63, 75, 77, 132, 138, 173–175, 178; role in polio therapy, 25, 74, 90, 98–101, 117, 121. *See also* serum

bloodletting, *see* therapies
boards of health, *see* health departments
Bodian, David, 175
Bolduan, Charles F., 38, 156
Boston Children's Hospital, 173, 175
Brodie, Maurice, 171. *See also* vaccines, polio
Brues, Charles, 61–63, 151–153
Burnet, F. Macfarlane, 177
Bussey Institute, 62, 151

Cantor, Eddie, 170
Carrick, Manton M., 9–10, 19
carriers: of disease, 139, 144; of polio, 5, 21, 28–36, 46–47, 50, 62, 98, 141, 144, 148, 150, 153, 190, 204n99. *See also* dust; food; immigrants; insects; Typhoid Mary
Carter, Richard, 184
Catt, Carrie Chapman, 68
Caverly, Charles S., 141
Centers for Disease Control (CDC), 180
Chapin, Charles V., 16, 46, 50, 58, 129, 159
Chicago Tribune, 101
children: polio as illness of, 1, 101, 124, 130, 157, 165; as research subjects, 80, 99, 175–178, 180, 185; at risk of polio, 6, 30–33, 36, 39, 43, 47, 49, 52–53, 57, 62–71, 118, 129, 131, 133, 146, 150, 156, 160, 188; sick, 66, 87, 96, 108, 144; vaccinated, 177–178, 185; as victims of polio, 1–2, 19, 36–42, 50, 63, 70, 77, 84–86, 91–93, 108, 110, 114, 117, 122, 127–128, 141–142, 146, 148, 152–155, 158–159, 162, 165–166, 170, 172
chiropractic, 102, 118
cholera, 2, 15, 31, 56, 61, 73, 77, 129, 139, 157
churches, 40, 55; Sunday schools, 40, 55–56
Cincinnati, University of, 181
city, the, 37, 132, 135–136; associated with polio, 31, 33, 142–145, 152, 165, 188, 190; dangers of, 30,

47, 49, 71, 124–125, 129, 131; as target of reform, 19, 57, 69, 123, 137, 139, 144–145. *See also* Progressive reform
City College of New York, 179
cleanliness, *see* sanitation
clergy, 33, 40, 56, 58, 134. *See also* William Harvey Young
Cobb, Stanley, 160
Coleman, William, 143
College of Physicians and Surgeons of New York, 94
Collins, Joseph, 141, 147
Columbia University, 26
counterirritation, *see* therapies
Cox, Herald, 180–182. *See also* vaccines, polio
Crippler, The (polio film), 171
Crowe, John, 92
Cushing, Harvey, 92
Cutter incident, 180, 182–184, 186, 188

Davis, Nancy, 171
de Kruif, Paul, 171–172, 178, 181, 183
department stores, 5, 64
diagnostic tests, 17–18, 72–74, 78–79, 154; for polio, 24–25, 28, 38, 44, 73–89, 92, 95, 98, 103–104, 107, 123, 139–144, 158–159, 163. *See also* blood; lumbar puncture; Schick test; Wasserman test; Widal test
diphtheria, 15, 17, 28, 73–74, 78, 86–89, 96, 98, 102, 117, 122, 129, 190n2. *See also* antitoxins; Schick test
dirt: role in disease, 3–4, 6–7, 13, 18–19, 29, 57, 107, 125, 129, 132–133, 137, 139, 143, 158; role in polio, 5, 8–10, 19, 31–33, 41, 43, 46–47, 52, 55, 60, 63–67, 70–71, 125–126, 144–145, 150–156, 162, 164, 169, 188–190
disability, 1, 101, 166, 168–169, 172, 176–177, 180, 187
disease, 3–8, 11, 15–18, 21, 31–34, 52, 55, 58, 60, 66, 69, 73, 77, 80,

82, 98–99, 109, 123, 129–137, 143, 158–159, 163, 166, 188–190, anthrax, 61, 129; arthritis, 188; Bright's disease, 114; dysentery, 17, 61; encephalitis, 173; eczema, 112; gastroenteritis, 77, 87; gonorrhea, 17; hookworm, 18, 155; mumps, 176; rheumatism, 77; scarlet fever, 31, 124, 157; sleeping sickness, 128, 139; spotted fever, 128; tonsillitis, 77, 104; typhus, 84, 139; venereal disease 122, 152, 232n17. *See also* cholera; diphtheria; influenza; malaria; measles; meningitis; plague; pneumonia; polio; rabies; smallpox; syphilis; tetanus; tuberculosis; typhoid fever; whooping cough; yellow fever

disinfectants: polio preventative, 18–19, 44, 46, 60, 75, 93, 101, 103, 117, 125–126; polio therapy, 89, 92–97, 101, 114, 117, 121–122; polio therapy: hexamethylenamin (urotropin), 92–93, 97, 120; polio therapy: hydrogen peroxide, 120

Dixon, Samuel Gibson, 26, 35, 39, 58, 63, 66

Dochez, Alphonse Raymond, 75–76

Doty, Alvah H., 158–159, 163

Dowling, Harry, 184

Draper, George, 75–76

Drinker respirators, *see* iron lung machines

drugs, *see* therapies

DuBois, Phebe, 81, 83–84, 94, 98

dust: role in disease, 129, 132, 136; role in polio, 53, 58, 70, 139, 150 151, 158

education, health, as polio preventative, 3, 19, 32, 38–40, 43, 50–57, 67, 69, 96, 103, 130, 151, 158–159. *See also* films; flies; New York City Bureau of Health Education; sanitation

Eisenhower, Dwight, 180, 183

Emerson, Haven: anti-polio campaign, 36, 43, 52, 62–63, 96, 99, 107–108, 148, 190; career, 26; efforts to explain polio, 50, 155–157; relations with public, 19, 34, 39–41, 53, 55, 64, 70, 78, 107, 113, 118–121, 124–125

Enders, John F., 24, 173, 175–177, 180, 188

entomology, *see* medical entomology

epidemiologists, in polio research, 6, 11, 26–28, 48, 58, 63, 76, 110, 144–147, 150, 154, 165, 174, 183, 188–189. *See also* Allen W. Freeman, Wade H. Frost, John R. Paul, Ivar Wickman

epidemiology, 27, 139, 140–141, 166; of polio, 5–7, 13, 19, 28, 55, 57, 61, 66, 71, 75, 77, 98, 107, 124–125, 131–132, 138–164, 190

Felt, Ephraim, 62

Fighting Infantile Paralysis (polio film) 10, 22–23, 52

films, 19, 32, 52, 171. *See also The Crippler, Fighting Infantile Paralysis*

filth, *see* dirt

filth theory of disease, 16, 18–19, 56, 60, 70, 144, 151, 157, 159

Fleming, Alexander, 176

Flexner, Simon: as laboratory researcher, 25, 76–79, 84–87, 90, 94–97; as polio expert, 20–22, 28, 50, 54, 63, 70, 101, 107–108, 112–117, 121, 125, 134–135, 160; as polio researcher, 23–24, 76, 81–82, 93, 98, 159; theory of polio, 23–24, 62, 76–79, 88, 110, 130, 138, 144, 154, 160–161, 173–175, 181

flies: as disease carriers, 19, 33; as target of anti-polio campaigns, 5, 9–10, 19–21, 26, 33, 55, 57–70, 101, 103, 126–128, 133, 136, 144, 150–154, 189–190; black fly, 128; housefly, 19, 59–64; stable fly, 61–64, 128, 158

Florida State Board of Health, 25

fomites (inanimate objects), 58, 70, 139

food: role in disease, 4, 25, 54; role
  in polio, 19, 53, 55, 58, 64–69,
  118, 124–133, 136–137, 157, 161,
  164
Francis, Thomas, Jr., 177, 179–180
Freeman, Allen W., 140, 146–148,
  160, 162
Frost, Wade H., 27, 62, 81, 95, 140,
  146–147, 151, 153, 161
Fulton, John S., 157

garbage: role in disease, 16, 18, 133,
  156; role in polio, 10, 46–47, 52–
  55, 64–69, 132
gay rights, 6
germ theory of disease, 3–8, 15–18,
  28–32, 46, 58, 60, 70, 89, 109,
  117, 122, 135–139, 142, 157, 163,
  190
germs: as agents of disease, 4, 8, 10,
  14–15, 18–22, 25, 29, 32, 44, 49,
  60–61, 66, 107, 117, 122–123,
  132, 136, 144, 153, 155, 162, 164,
  173, 188; in laboratory, 74, 78,
  82–83, 87–88, 97, 104, 109–110,
  173. *See also* virus
German immigrants, *see* immigrants

Hamilton, Alice, 60
handicap, *see* disability
Harvard Medical School, 26, 140,
  154, 175; researchers, 150
Harvard-MIT School for Health Officers, 26, 140
Hatch, Edward, Jr., 64
Hayes, Helen, 107
health certificates, in anti-polio campaigns, 36–38
health departments, 11, 16–18, 25,
  32, 78, 96, 125, 140. *See also* U.S.
  Public Health Service
health education, *see* education
health officials, 4, 26–28, 103–106,
  123, 189–190, 124, 145; anti-fly
  campaigns of, 57–69, 128, 154;
  and immigrants, 19, 21, 42–43,
  49–50; and polio, 3, 5–6, 10–11,
  13–14, 26–44, 69–71, 86, 95–101,
  109–110, 139, 150, 155–157,

160–163, 175–178; and sanitation, 4, 6, 44–57, 136, 139; federal, 36, 43, 146–148, 179–180,
  186; in Massachusetts, 61, 92, 140,
  151, 153–154; in Minnesota, 77,
  93, 140, 150; in New Jersey, 36,
  39–43, 53, 64, 157, 159; in New
  York City, 13, 35–36, 63, 67, 79,
  86, 93–99, 126, 140, 142, 148,
  152, 156, 158, 160; in New York
  State, 35–36, 41, 67, 147; in Pennsylvania, 35, 39–40, 48; in Philadelphia, 36, 38, 41, 43, 48–49, 53,
  55, 96. *See also* Hermann Biggs;
  Haven Emerson; Wade H. Frost;
  Wilmer Krusen
Heine, Jacob, 141
Henry Phipps Institute laboratory,
  86
hexamethylenamin (urotropin), *see*
  disinfectants
Hill, Herbert Winslow, 77–78, 93,
  140, 150–151
Hobby, Oveta Culp, 180
Holt, Luther Emmett, 86–87
homeopathy, 49
Horstmann, Dorothy M., 174
hospitals, 33, 55, 62, 72–81, 85–86,
  94–99, 103–104, 110, 160–161;
  for children, 39–41, 173, 175. *See
  also* Boston Children's Hospital;
  Johns Hopkins Hospital; Kingston Avenue Hospital; Queens Borough Hospital for Contagious Disease; Rockefeller Institute for
  Medical Research; Smith Infirmary
housefly, *see* flies
Howard, L. O., 61
Howard, William Schley, 47
Howe, Howard, 175
hydropathy, 118, 168
hygiene, *see* sanitation
Hygienic Laboratory (of U.S. Public
  Health Service), 58, 62, 95, 152,
  154

immigrants: and disease, 10, 19, 21,
  29–32, 46–47, 125, 128, 145, 148,

150, 159; and polio, 1, 3–4, 8, 19–
20, 29–33, 42, 46–49, 54, 57, 70,
86, 123, 125, 136, 143–144, 148–
150, 156–157, 163–166, 169,
188–189; Eastern European, 3,
14, 47, 144, 147, 190; English,
144; German, 15, 47, 114, 148;
Irish, 15, 47, 114, 144, 148; Italian, 15, 19, 41–42, 47, 54, 132,
148, 150, 156, 202n58; Jewish, 11,
19, 47, 156, 181; Polish, 47, 50,
148, 155–156; Russian, 15, 47,
148; Slavic, 47, 150
infant health stations, 54, 155–156
infantile paralysis, *see* polio
influenza, 119, 131–132, 177
insects: as disease carriers, 18–19,
28, 54, 60, 128, 139, 154; as polio
carriers, 19–21, 58–59, 63–64,
127, 129, 143–145, 150–154, 161,
164; bedbugs, 61, 116, 128–129,
150, 152–153; cockroaches, 59,
128–129; fleas, 59, 63, 152, 158;
hookworm, 18; lice, 59, 128; nits,
44; tarantulas, 127. *See also* flies;
mosquitoes
International Congress on Hygiene
and Demography (1912), 61–62
Irish immigrants, *see* immigrants
iron lung machines, 1, 176
Italian immigrants, *see* immigrants

Jews, *see* immigrants
Johns Hopkins Hospital, 92
Johns Hopkins Medical School, 21;
researchers, 157, 160, 177
Johns Hopkins School of Public
Health and Hygiene, 26–27, 140
*Journal of the American Medical Associa-
tion (JAMA)*, 60, 63, 82, 85, 90, 93,
98

Kansas State Board of Health, 25
Keen, William Williams, 167
Kenny, Elizabeth, 176, 187; Kenny
Foundation, 176, 181
Kingston Avenue Hospital (New
York), 42, 94
Klein, Aaron, 183, 188

Koch, Robert, 3, 14, 22; Koch Insti-
tute, 22
Kolmer, John, 171
Koprowski, Hilary, 180, 182. *See also*
vaccines, polio
Krusen, Wilmer, 43, 53, 66–67, 96

laboratory, 3–7, 17–18, 25–28, 72–
74, 78–79, 96, 109, 139, 177,
183–184, 189; use in polio research, 3, 5, 19, 24–25, 28, 71–77,
83–90, 95–98, 103–105, 112,
116–117, 120, 135, 139, 151, 154,
159, 168, 174, 178, 180, 190. *See
also* Henry Phipps Institute laboratory; Hygienic Laboratory;
Lederle Laboratories; Rockefeller
Institute for Medical Research
Landsteiner, Karl, 23, 98
Lavinder, Claude, 147
Leavitt, Judith Walzer, 108
Lederle Laboratories, 180. *See also*
vaccines, polio
Levaditi, Constanin, 23, 98
Lewis, Paul, 86, 93, 98
Lovett, Robert W., 140, 160, 167
lumbar puncture: for polio diagnosis, 25, 74, 79–87, 103, 120, 167;
for polio therapy, 93–94, 103, 167

McAdoo, William G., 159
MacLean, Alistair, 182
malaria, 17, 59, 61, 128, 139, 151
March of Dimes, *see* National Foun-
dation for Infantile Paralysis
Massachusetts State Board of
Health, 61, 140
Mayer, Edward, 83, 85
measles, 2, 31, 124, 146, 157, 198n2
medical entomology, 4, 18–19, 59–
64, 128, 139, 144, 150–151. *See
also* Charles Brues; Ephraim Felt;
L. O. Howard
medical journals, 26, 108, 118, 131.
*See also American Journal of Diseases
of Children; American Journal of
Electrotherapeutics and Radiology;
American Journal of Public Health;
Journal of the American Medical Asso-*

medical journals (*continued*)
  *ciation; Medical Record; New York
  Medical Journal; New York State Journal of Medicine*
Medical Record, 158
medical sectarians, 118. *See also* chiropractic; homeopathy;
  hydropathy; Thomsonianism
Meltzer, Simon J., 94, 97
meningitis, 17, 22, 77, 81–87, 94–
  97. *See also* serum
Michigan, University of, 177
milk: dangers of pasteurization,
  124–125, 137, 155; role in disease,
  22, 25; role in polio, 118, 124–
  126, 136, 143, 157–159, 164
Minnesota State Board of Health,
  140. *See also* Herbert Winslow Hill
Minnesota, University of, 176
Mitchel, John P., 72, 107, 118, 124,
  132–134
monkeys: as laboratory subjects in
  polio research, 5, 23–24, 61, 75–
  76, 79, 82, 87–89, 95, 98–100,
  103, 116, 138, 174–175; Rhesus
  monkeys, 23–24, 82, 168, 174
mosquitoes: as disease carriers, 52;
  role in malaria, 59; role in polio,
  127–128; role in yellow fever, 18,
  28, 59. *See also* Walter Reed; Ronald Ross
mothers, *see* women
Motion Picture Exhibitors League,
  42. *See also* films
movie theaters, 5, 32, 42–43, 53, 57
movies, *see* films

National Academy of Sciences, 185
National Foundation for Infantile Paralysis, 166, 170–171, 180, 187–
  188; Birthday Balls, 170–171;
  March of Dimes campaign, 1,
  170–171, 188; publicity, 166, 172,
  179, 183, 185, 188; role in polio
  research, 166, 171–173, 176–177,
  181, 184, 186; role in vaccine trials, 178–182
National Institutes of Health, 178
National Tuberculosis Association,
  172

nativism, 47, 144, 148. *See also* immi-
  grants
Neal, Josephine, 81–84, 94, 98
neurologists, 92, 141–142
New Jersey State Department of
  Health, 42
New Public Health, 16, 18–19, 30–
  71, 129, 144, 150, 158, 163, 189.
  See also germ theory of disease
New York Academy of Medicine, 50,
  63
New York City Bureau of Health
  Education, 38, 52, 156
New York City Department of
  Health, 11, 26, 36, 40, 42, 81, 93,
  98, 118, 126, 132, 135, 140, 151–
  152; laboratories, 79, 83, 86, 96–
  97. *See also* Harry L. Abramson;
  Phebe DuBois; Haven Emerson;
  Josephine Neal
New York City Department of Street
  Cleaning, 52, 126
New York Medical Journal, 94
New York Merchants Association,
  Fly-Fighting Committee, 64
New York Society for the Prevention
  of Cruelty to Animals, 59
New York State Department of
  Health, 34, 58. *See also* Hermann
  Biggs
New York State Journal of Medicine, 153
New York State Medical Society, 84
New York Times, 21–22, 30, 48, 50,
  66, 94, 130, 135
New York University, 177; College of
  Medicine, 179, 181
Newark Evening News, 128
Newark Department of Public
  Health, 40, 157
newspapers: polio reports, 25, 34,
  42–43, 48, 52–56, 62, 65, 67, 72,
  101, 106, 115–116, 123, 131, 134.
  *See also Chicago Tribune; New York
  Times; Newark Evening News; Phila-
  delphia Evening Bulletin; Philadel-
  phia Inquirer*
Noguchi, Hideyo, 21, 23–24, 78,
  82–83, 159
nurses, 11, 49–50, 54, 111, 113. *See
  also* Elizabeth Kenny

nutrition, 172, 176, 187. *See also* food

O'Connor, D. Basil, 166, 171, 176, 178, 187
Osler, William, 92

Page, Walter Hines, 48
Park, William Hallock, 159, 171. *See also* vaccines, polio
paralysis, *see* polio
parents: anxious, 41, 49, 58, 91, 133; and child care, 46, 71, 130–131, 162; fear of polio, 19, 32, 165; protection of children, 34, 40–42, 44, 53, 68–69, 76, 86, 108, 130, 142, 144, 148, 152, 154, 160, 188
Pasteur, Louis, 3, 14, 97, 100, 103, 176; Pasteur Institute, 21, 98
pasteurization, *see* milk
pathologists, 73, 80–84, 86, 94, 98–99, 103–105
pathology, 74, 78, 116, 118
patients, 107–108, 120; with polio, 25, 28, 44, 47, 58, 61, 72–75, 79–94, 97, 99, 102–104, 113, 135, 141, 154, 160, 168, 170, 176; role in polio research, 79, 83, 95, 116, 118, 175
Paul, John R., 88, 174, 179, 183, 186–187
Peabody, Francis, 75–76
peddlers, role in polio, 130, 157
pediatricians, 86, 94, 140–142. *See also* Luther Emmett Holt
Pennsylvania State Department of Health, 35. *See also* Samuel Gibson Dixon
Philadelphia Board of Recreation, 49
Philadelphia Department of Public Health, 41. *See also* Wilmer Krusen
Philadelphia Evening Bulletin, 48
Philadelphia Housing Association, 52
Philadelphia Inquirer, 132
Pittsburgh, University of, 177
placards, 37, 39, 47

playgrounds, 40, 42, 49, 59
physicians, 79, 90, 108, 120; and insect theory, 18, 144, 153–154; and the laboratory, 18, 25, 72–74, 80–86; and lay healers, 113–115, 119, 176, 187; and polio, 5, 7, 11, 13, 19, 21, 25, 28–31, 37–40, 46–49, 53, 55, 58–60, 69, 75–81, 85, 88–93, 94–96, 99, 103, 107–111, 121–125, 128, 137, 142, 157–160, 162, 165–166, 170, 182, 189; as polio carriers, 44–45, 49–50, 62, 155; as polio experts, 4, 129, 132, 135; and polio therapies, 99–104; as researchers, 26, 82, 140, 145, 153, 185. *See also* health officials
plague, 73, 77, 129, 132, 139, 152
pneumonia, 17, 77, 96, 116, 119, 121
polio: epidemic of 1916, 5–6, 9–14, 21–22, 25–29, 30–72, 76, 80–81, 90, 93–99, 106–111, 117–120, 124–129, 135, 137, 140–141, 146–147, 151–162, 190; epidemics, 1–3, 5–6, 10–11, 18, 28–31, 42, 53, 58, 76–79, 86, 89, 106–110, 123, 132, 140–148, 150–154, 161–162, 165–166, 170, 178, 186, 189–190; histories of, 182–188; image of, 1, 142, 165–167, 188; immunity to, 2, 18, 24, 89, 95, 98, 166, 173–181, 186; intestinal model of, 24, 160–161, 165, 173–175, 181; neurological model of, 23–24, 44, 50, 75–79, 82, 89, 92, 130, 138, 141, 161, 165; and paralysis, 1, 23, 38, 48, 59, 75, 77–81, 84–87, 93, 101–103, 114, 120, 141–148, 158, 163–167, 174–176, 179–181, 186; publicity, 44, 101, 106, 170–172, 179, 185; rehabilitation, 170; research, 5, 13, 22–23, 75, 81, 166, 171–176, 189; symptoms, 2, 11, 23, 28, 53, 61–62, 75–77, 84–95, 98, 104, 110, 115, 120–122, 141–144, 147, 158–167, 174–175. *See also* diagnostic tests; National Foundation for Infantile Paralysis; therapies; virus
Polish immigrants, *see* immigrants

post-polio syndrome, 189
Progressive reform, 4, 14–15, 57,
  134; and health reform, 15, 17,
  124; and role of science, 4, 14–15,
  28, 32, 72; and urban reform, 14,
  42–43, 69, 144
public: fear of dirt, 31, 60, 67, 159;
  fear of flies, 56, 64, 67–68; fear of
  polio, 3, 19, 30, 36, 38, 42, 46, 49,
  55, 58, 157, 172, 178; faith in science, 5, 28, 30, 72–73, 96, 100–
  102, 109, 113, 116–117, 135, 172,
  178–179, 182–186, 188; and lay
  healers, 29, 106–107, 111–115,
  119–123, 190; and polio, 6, 28–
  29, 31, 37–40, 70, 72, 77, 106–
  137, 187, 189; suspicion of science, 6, 22, 25, 118, 135
public health, see health officials;
  New Public Health; sanitary science

quarantine: against AIDS, 7; against
  polio, 5–6, 11, 30–44, 56, 67, 81,
  106, 110, 157–158
Queens Borough Hospital for Contagious Diseases, 44

rabies, 17–18, 22, 73, 97
race, as factor in polio, 13, 111, 168
Raskob, John H., 169
Reed, Walter, 18, 28, 59–60, 151
Rivers, Thomas M., 24, 180
Robbins, Frederick, 173
Rockefeller, John D., Jr., 21, 107,
  112, 114; Rockefeller Foundation,
  106–107, 112, 158
Rockefeller Institute for Medical Research, 5, 21–23, 50, 52, 93, 101,
  104, 107, 116, 118, 135, 181; Hospital, 75–76; polio research, 24,
  75–79, 88, 93–94, 97, 110, 112–
  117, 122, 138, 140. See also Simon
  Flexner, Hideyo Noguchi
Roosevelt, Eleanor, 167–168, 187
Roosevelt, Franklin Delano: as polio
  victim, 1, 140, 167; support polio
  research, 171; as symbol of polio,
  1, 3, 166, 169, 179, 187–188, 190;

therapy of, 167–168. See also Na-
  tional Foundation for Infantile Pa-
  ralysis; Warm Springs
Rosenau, Milton J., 26, 61–62, 140,
  150
Rosenberg, Charles, 120
Ross, Ronald, 18, 39, 151
Russian immigrants, see immigrants

Sabin, Albert, 177–182, 186–187
Sabin vaccine, see vaccines, polio
Sachs, Bernard, 142
Salk, Jonas E., 175, 177–185, 188–
  189; Salk Institute for Biological
  Studies, 185
Salk vaccine, see vaccines, polio
sanitary products, as polio preventative, 44, 52, 129
sanitary science, 16, 18, 31–33, 57,
  60, 139, 157. See also filth theory
  of disease
sanitation, 2, 6, 16, 19, 139, 144–
  146, 150, 165; as polio preventative, 30, 32, 57, 96, 126, 132, 136,
  158–163, 189–190; public health
  campaigns for, 4–6, 19, 44–50,
  52–56, 60, 63–70, 155–156, 161;
  role of, in polio epidemiology,
  103, 125–130, 132, 143, 147, 154,
  166
Scheele, Leonard A., 180
Schick test (for diphtheria), 17, 98
schools, 40, 189
scientists, 22, 24, 86, 108, 116–118,
  134; and debate on polio, 3, 72,
  88, 107; in polio research, 2–5,
  25–28, 32, 50, 53, 58, 61, 64, 67,
  70, 75–83, 90, 97, 99, 104, 106,
  110, 115, 120, 122, 138–139, 144,
  160, 165–167, 170–173, 176–178,
  183–189; role in National Foundation, 166–167, 170–173
sera, 16–17, 74, 96, 135; anti-
  meningitis, 95–97, 101; for measles, 99; for pneumonia, 96
serum, anti-polio, 25, 74–75, 94–
  104, 117, 178, 190; gamma
  globulin, 178; normal, 95–102; recovered, 74, 98–101

Sheppard, Philip, 61, 159
Simmons, George H., 90
Slavic immigrants, see immigrants
smallpox, 17, 22, 31, 38, 61, 102, 158
Smith, Alfred E., 169, 188
Smith, Jane, 184–185
Smith Infirmary (New York), 160
Snow, William Benham, 93–94
social workers, 34–35, 42, 54–55, 69
South Carolina State Board of Medical Examiners, 90
spinal tap, see lumbar puncture
Starr, Paul, 28
Staten Island Civic League, 67, 133
Straus, Nathan, 124
swimming pools, role in polio, 1, 29, 167, 197n60. See also water
syphilis, 15, 17–18, 74, 77, 83, 154, 198n2. See also Wassermann test

Taylor, Zachary, 134
tetanus, 17, 73, 96, 116. See also antitoxins
therapies, for polio, 19, 56, 73–75, 88–105, 107, 110, 119–123, 139, 160, 166–167, 176, 189; alcohol, 120; adrenalin, 94–96; bloodletting, 89, 91, 120–122, 137; camphor, 114; chemical, 91, 113, 119–122; counterirritation, 89, 92, 121, 137; diphtheria antitoxin, 117; herbs, 113, 116, 119; hot packs, 91; massage, 121, 167; nasal spray, 93, 175; purgatives, 91, 114, 137; salves, 115–116, 119, 121–123. See also disinfectants; lumbar puncture; serum; water
Thomsonianism, 116
tuberculosis (consumption), 15, 61, 74, 77–78, 81, 114–115, 119–120, 124, 129–130, 157, 198n2. See also National Tuberculosis Association
Tuskegee Institute, and polio rehabilitation, 169
typhoid fever, 2, 15, 17, 31, 56, 60–61, 66, 73–74, 77–78, 81, 87, 96, 102, 124, 139, 154, 157, 161. See also Widal test
Typhoid Mary, 36, 144

U.S. Public Health Service: and polio, 36–37, 78, 124; and polio epidemiology, 11, 140, 146–147, 151; and polio research, 25–26, 62, 173. See also John F. Anderson; Allen W. Freeman; Wade H. Frost; Hygienic Laboratory

vaccination, see anti-vaccination movement; vaccines
vaccines, 16, 73–74, 96–97, 102, 117, 135–136, 158; for AIDS, 6, 189
vaccines, polio, 1–2, 166, 176–183, 189–190; Brodie-Park, 171, 183; Koprowski, 182; Lederle-Cox, 181; Sabin (live-virus), 171, 177, 179–182, 186, 188; Salk (killed-virus), 171, 177–179, 183–184, 186, 188; trials of, 171, 175, 178 181, 186, 188
virologists, polio, 24–25, 76, 140, 165, 172–173, 176, 179–180, 189. See also John F. Enders; Simon Flexner
virology, 22–25, 77, 154, 166, 176, 189
virus, polio, 22–25, 28, 48, 50, 61, 63, 68, 74–78, 93, 100, 104, 126–127, 130–131, 154–155, 159, 161, 188; research on, 75–79, 82, 88, 95, 98–99, 110–111, 138–139, 141, 171–175, 180–181; strains of, 24, 165, 173–176, 179; virulence, 138, 165, 180

Warm Springs, Georgia, 168–169, 187
wars: Spanish-American, 60; World War I, 13–14, 133, 183; World War II, 174–178, 184
Washington Market Merchants Association (New York), 64
Wassermann test (for syphilis), 17, 217n113
water: as polio cause, 131, 166, 168; as polio preventative, 52, 160, 202n56; as polio therapy, 117–118, 120–121, 134, 166–168; role

water (*continued*)
  in disease, 4, 25, 54, 69, 139, 157.
  See also hydropathy; swimming
  pools; Warm Springs
Weaver, Harry, 176–178, 186
Weller, Thomas, 173
Wickman, Ivar, 77, 141–146, 158,
  163
Widal test (for typhoid), 17, 87
Winchell, Walter, 178
Winslow, C.-E. A., 155, 161
whooping cough, 17, 31, 157
women, 33, 41, 48, 58–59, 67, 153,
  187; as housekeepers, 9, 15, 18–
  19, 52–53, 55, 111, 117, 119, 125–
  129, 158–159, 161; as mothers, 11,
  30, 33, 40–42, 47, 52, 55, 66–67,
  85, 91, 101, 111, 114–116, 118,
  121, 124–125, 129–130, 156; as reformers, 15, 33, 68–69; as suffragists, 68–69, 132; suggest polio
  causes, 111, 117–118, 125–128,
  132, 134; suggest polio therapies,
  106–107, 111–117, 120–122; as
  teachers, 53, 117. *See also* nurses;
  pathologists; social workers
World Health Organization, 181

Yale Poliomyelitis Unit, 174–175
yellow fever, 18, 22, 28, 31, 59, 61,
  63, 73, 121, 128, 139, 143, 151–
  152, 158
Young, William Harvey, 33, 40, 58

Zingher, Abraham, 99–102